ZEN

in Motion

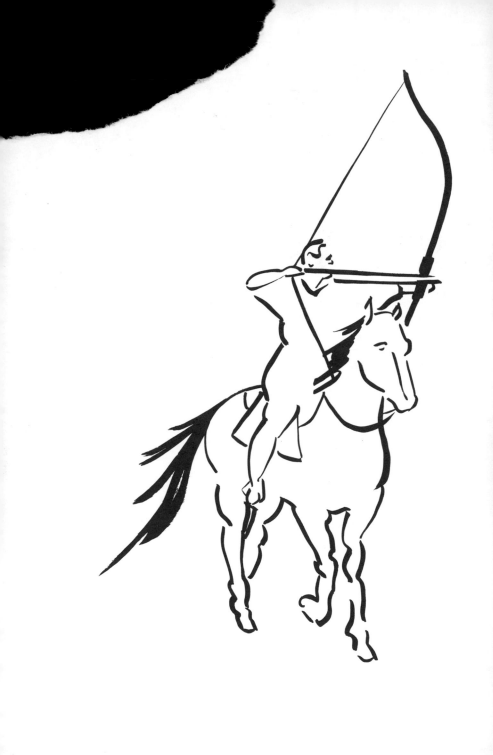

Z in Motion
ZEN

**LESSONS FROM
A MASTER ARCHER
ON BREATH,
POSTURE,
AND THE PATH OF
INTUITION**

NEIL CLAREMON

Inner Traditions International
Rochester, Vermont

Inner Traditions International, Ltd.
One Park Street
Rochester, Vermont 05767

Copyright © 1991 Neil Claremon

Library of Congress Cataloging-in-Publication Data

Claremon, Neil.
  Zen in motion : lessons from a master archer on breath, posture, and the path of intuition / Neil Clarmon.
      p. cm.
  ISBN 0-89281-361-X (pbk.)
  1. Archery. 2. Archery—Psychological aspects. 3. Zen Buddhism. 4. Breathing exercises. 5. Posture. I. Title.
  GV1185.C42 1991
  799.3'2—dc20   91-28912
                                                                          CIP

Text design by Virginia L. Scott.
Illustrations on pages 88–96 by Ray Rue.
All other text illustrations by Michael John Martin Ridge.

Printed and bound in the United States

10   9   8   7   6   5   4   3   2   1

Distributed to the book trade in the United States by American International Distribution Corporation (AIDC) Publishers, Inc.

Distributed to the book trade in Canada by Book Center, Inc., Montreal, Quebec.

For my father and son.

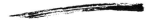

Thus shall ye think of all this fleeting world:
A star at dawn, a bubble in a stream;
A flash of lightning in a summer cloud,
A flickering lamp, a phantom, and a dream.

The Diamond Sutra

CONTENTS

INTRODUCTION
THE ARC OF KI

The practice of Zen is traditionally associated with stillness, even sedentariness. Yet its deepest roots may lie in the maximizing of survival skills attained by horsemen who had to hunt and fight with bows and arrows. Some of Zen's most paradoxical lessons derive from mastering motion.

When bows and arrows are linked to horses, we Americans usually think of the Lakota and Apache. A close examination of American Indian bows, however, quickly reveals their limitations, and it is very unlikely that they shot arrows on horseback from anything but close range. To rediscover the mastery of accuracy in motion, I had to turn to the traditions of the Far East and the disciplining of the intuitive ability through the cultivation of ki.

Ki is the Japanese word for what the Chinese call *chi,* the Hindus call *prana,* the Apache call *diyin,* the Pygmies call *mana.* In this book I use *ki* to mean the indwelling force. This force manifests as the feel of a direction or pattern frozen within an instant. A master of ki tells us that, in certain states, the mind sees the arc of this force in a flash of intuition. This way of knowing, the master says, depends on the subtle adjustments that occur with constant repetitions of form and on the consciousness that tells us when rather than how to do something. In other words, the intuitive faculty, although innate, must be trained and organized if it is to become reliable. A concentrated stance-attitude and a breath-controlled posture are the two chariots of the trained intuition. The more these two (which are inseparable in the long run) are disciplined, the more ki is available.

In the West physical action and the indwelling life force are rarely associated, but in the East they cannot be disassociated. The joining of physical ability with spiritual work is much like the combination of grace in action. That the means, the form, can be considered more important than the result is not only alien to most Westerners, it makes no sense at all in our systems. Since what is not readily comprehensible often makes us angry, we resist learning new coordinates of our inner selves. To circumvent such resistance, I will avoid any preaching in order to concentrate on the training derived from acting in accordance with ki. When I watch my teacher shoot his bow, I see his stance, his posture, his breathing, and his way of composing himself, rather than eight traditional steps for shooting a Japanese bow. I find that he walks with the same composure as he shoots his bow or rides his horse. As Eugen Herrigel suggests in *Zen in the Art of Archery,* the Japanese had turned the ancient practice of archery into a practice for living. A master's arrows penetrate deeper than a student's do, and his teachings change the personality of the archer along with the very idea of what the target is. The target is no longer an external object, the target *is* the archer.

In centuries past, a most complex training was reserved

for the Japanese nobility learning to shoot arrows from horseback. Having to deal with speed and aim simultaneously required a subtle teaching in what might be translated as "the path of intuition" or "the way of self-containment." The teaching was kept in the hands of a very few. The last to have received it in a traditional manner are now in their eighties, and the most advanced disciple presently living in the West is prone to solitude. Oddly, the teaching is even more necessary in this age of speed and motion than it was centuries ago as a means of self-defense: It is a perfect antidote to the hurry and stress of our time. The hard part of translating it from Japan to modern America is that cultivation of the ki belongs to a time when selflessness was valued, but it must be transmitted to an age steeped in the cult of personality.

In the Zen practice of archery, the bow string goes forward, the arrow releases, and, imitating the master, I groan-grunt-shout with the exertion. There is no word in English for the action-yell I experience, and the "I" that achieves it is stranger yet. In Japanese the word is *kiai*. It describes the exhalation of breath caused by the contraction of the abdominal muscles. The breath is forced through the vocal cords in a loud burst that releases air in an almost magical resonance with the string and the arrow. The breath follows the arrow and the arrow follows the breath as the archer becomes one with the Sea of Origin, the universal flux of matter and energy. In my experience, resonance with ki while in motion spells the difference between spiritual awareness and self-assertion. An arrow shot in alignment with ki is called a strong arrow. There is a qualitative difference between shooting an arrow when harmony is present and when it is absent that has nothing to do with right or wrong, good or bad, accurate or inaccurate. The difference is visible in the archer's demeanor; it is a kind of grace that is not attained for the sake of gracefulness.

My story is a description of this discipline that was lacking in my life because it was not available in the West. I was not looking for any specific training, nor did I have any intention of becoming a student. I went to visit a Zen archery center in the southwestern United States to see what more about ki could be learned from those who had been taught in the traditional manner. Despite many traumas, the center's school of instruction had survived the westernization of Japan. The traditional, hereditary master of this school of horseback archery had survived World War II. Both he and his main disciple lived for part of the year in the Rocky Mountains. I had been given an introduction to the younger disciple, who was known as being more eclectic and less regimented in his teachings than his own master.

My learning was informal, a training in taking responsibility for myself by improving my intuition and grasping the underlying arc of ki in the moment. I discovered that this grasp reached into many areas of my life beside archery. From the beginning, my affinity for the teacher gave me the willingness to make a long-term commitment to this school of Zen training. The surprise was in how far-reaching a transformation could come from taking lessons in breathing, posture, and the path of intuition.

In the West we tend to think of intuition as existing inside the head—as solely a mental thing—whereas in the

East the intuitive faculty can also be a physical attribute that resides primarily in the belly. My major shift in perspective depended on the realization that it was possible to train the physical intuition and thereby alter and improve my mental ability to intuit; that is, to sense complex situations simply. I learned that one can become more adept in the outside reality by better mastering the inner one. I no longer believe that the intuitive power resides in the head. I know it is an attribute of a well trained mind-body, and that learning new modes of breathing and aligning the body (posture) improves the ability to comprehend and to act in any situation.

To enhance a person's ideas about body, mind, and intuition, the Zen master brings the problem of shooting arrows from horseback along with a thousand years of tradition. Those who wish to change the composure at the center of their lives and improve the accuracy of their intuition will appreciate the revelations of this past.

1

PREPARATION

I went to the retreat on the mountain expecting to be taught how to develop my awareness of ki. The master's credentials were imposing, and I hoped he wouldn't refuse to teach me. Just watching him walk around was proof enough that he possessed the secret: even gravity didn't seem to be an obstacle for him. He didn't transcend it; he used it to walk with the contours of the land. Some of his students seemed blessed with the same agility. Here was a teacher who really taught, I felt. He wasn't bound by subject or style but had gone to the essence of what a person needed to know to be fully alive. The true mark of a master is the ability to sift out the extraneous and concentrate on the essentials, the moorings to which any other knowledge must be tied. It was a matter not of knowing how to move but of when to take the next step to catch the arc in the motion that corresponds to the existence of the much-investigated ki.

Everyone around the master knows that ki is not energy in the strict scientific sense. The usual translation of the Japanese character for ki is "the field of life." Most of the time we are unaware of this field, but every now and again something stuns our normal thoughts and provides us with a specific entrance into it.

Everyone at the retreat knew that ki was only measurable in its sudden presence. One of the older students demonstrated a simple technique for observing the ki within. He was a tall, gaunt monk with a chiselled face, who seemed to climb the steep mountain slope above the retreat without ever gasping for air. As graceful as the master, he, too, never seemed to strain at physical tasks. He had mastered a disciplined breathing rhythm that I would have to learn in due time. He asked me to press my ring finger into the palm of my hand. I bent it from the knuckle and pushed against the two lines going from my wrist into the center of my palm. "Do you feel anything?" he wanted to know. I repeated the procedure several times without feeling anything unusual. He walked around me twice and shook his head in dismay.

He suggested that I stand with a great deal more attention to my posture. What he meant by good posture surprised me, since his own posture was somewhat sway-backed. Using his rather large hands, he forced the small of my back inward. He pressed down on my shoulders, causing my belly to protrude, and told me to inhale through my nose, then blow my breath out through my mouth. At the split second before the breath was exhausted I was to press my ring finger into my palm.

I could barely mount much finger pressure when so nearly out of breath. What I could manage produced a kind of numb jar to my arm. It was a subtle feeling, although not so subtle that I couldn't recognize it as a minor version of what happens whenever I hit my funny bone. I had never suspected that this feeling was a relative of the much-touted ki, another kind of vibration in the nerves.

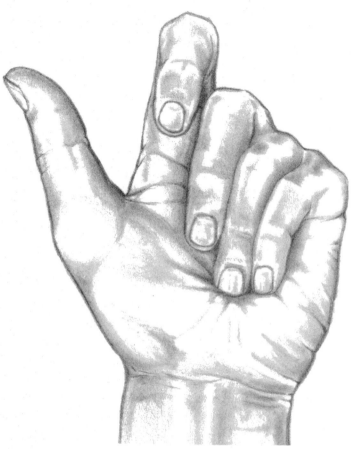

The sensitive area below the ring finger is a powerful spot for stimulating awareness of the ki energy's lines of force.

At that moment I was standing on a weathered rail tie that held up an embankment of dirt. It was a summer day with a high blue sky dotted with puffy white clouds. Blues and greens dominated the landscape. In a few seconds, many thoughts raced through my mind. I wondered why I had a preference about where ki should be and what it should or shouldn't feel like. I realized I was prejudicing myself against whatever happened to be.

The instant I concentrated on the point where my finger met the palm of my hand, a slight jolt shot up to my shoulder. Although the action of ki is too much to digest at first, I was willing to accept that it was indeed a force existing inside me. I could describe it specifically without reference to any religion or tradition. I could even imagine a method of walking that would produce a sensation in my legs comparable to this numb line of force in my arm with its magnetlike twinge of repelling polarities. I felt elated, even though all I had done was press my ring finger into my hand while standing a certain way and, as he had suggested, blow my breath through my lips and expand my belly.

He had about fifty seconds to observe me while I tried his little experiment. "You see," he said, "you didn't get there by knowing how to press your finger into your palm, but by waiting until the right instant, when it was possible to follow the arc of ki up your arm." It was obvious to him, yet up until a minute ago I hadn't had the slightest idea of it. In fact, I'd had the sensation many times before without knowing what it was or having a reason to cultivate it. I had felt the jolt when I shot an arrow and the twang of the release had reverberated through my body. With hindsight, I can say that this occurred only when I felt the perfection of the shot and knew it was going to be the one to hit the mark.

"What you just experienced," he continued, "has to do

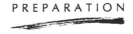

with the way your body cells line up with the universal flux around you. The breathing controls the nerve energy that determines the neurochemistry of the cells. A fuller breath makes the cells more vibrant."

This comment added a metaphysical dimension to my experience. The tone of his voice suggested that he meant a very orderly and controlled version of what for me had been an accidental event. An orderly version surely would allow more awareness of discrete actions. Slow motion could always be achieved by the way I was breathing— and by consequently lowering my center of attention from my eyes to my belly. Such a shift of perspective is like the throwing of a switch. All the tension and pressure that usually accumulate in the head dissipates, and greater bodily awareness, balance, and calmness are the result.

After exploring desert Native American practices for many years, I knew enough to equate spiritual work with the experience of expanded time. With the pressing of my finger into the lower part of my palm came the same calm alertness that goes with being immersed within great expanses and vistas. With this sense of space and time I knew I was close to the common Western idea of a spiritual experience: something that takes the breath away. I hadn't yet delved deeply enough to discover that the experience is multidimensional in the sense of being as physical as it is spiritual. In expanded time, lines of force seem to hold the body upright without any intentional action. One is both overwhelmed and inspired.

I'd had brief, accidental encounters of this kind, but the master felt that occasional contact with the field of life didn't provide a satisfactory way of living. The essential bearing he sought demanded nearly constant awareness, a continuous presence in mind. Remembering to press the ring finger into my palm before shooting an arrow was a simple way to remind myself that archery is a means of contacting the ubiquitous field of life. To make this contact I needed to aim through the center of the target and align with the full arc of the shot. This is both a literal and figurative rule. An arrow is much like a thought: useless if it doesn't penetrate to the heart of the matter. A master of penetration might be a monastic Zen Buddhist or a wood-cutter aware of the field of life at all times—the spirit of the Zen arrow didn't care which.

2

GROUNDING

Through friends I'd heard that the master lived in the Rockies in a spot that reminded him of the ranges above Kyoto. Three years passed before I was ready to visit him; meanwhile, I'd remained content with my life. This contentment often turned into overconfidence; there were many times when my resolutions to improve faltered. For the most part I ignored the inner doubts, but when my archery practice reached a new plateau of accuracy, I mustered the courage to face this disciple of a man who was considered the highest master of the art in his country.

I arrived at the center in the afternoon, as a sun shower pelted the road between rows of pine and fir trees. Driving through muddy ruts strewn with rocks, I arrived at a large stone building. No one was inside, but I heard an intermittent thudding, as if apples were falling. After a while four men and a woman came down the trail carrying long Japanese bows. They greeted me and invited me to wait for the master inside. These people were students and teachers. The master was out riding his horse but was due back shortly.

From the upper deck of the house I could see the cleared fields of an Indian pueblo. I heard horses whinnying in the pasture along the road. On one hillside a man in a Japanese robe was riding an Indian Paint and shooting bamboo arrows from a Mongolian saddle. I feared that he'd lost track of time. When he finally arrived, he greeted me politely, his manner almost deferential, and we spoke about our mutual friends. There was a guest cabin where I could stay, and he led me to it through the woods along a stream. I followed this slightly built, buoyant fifty-year-old man along the trail to where I was staying and intentionally imitated his footsteps, only to find that the best I could manage was an awkward improvisation. As I unpacked I showed him my short take-down bow, and he nodded but said nothing about shooting with him. The very serenity of his face—which was plain-featured except for unusually well developed muscles around the mouth—made any further suggestion impossible.

My bow remained in its case for many days. Before I'd left home, friends had asked me why I wanted to work on something so solitary as archery. I had a difficult time explaining why. We each have our own calling, and it's hard to explain it to another. The bow is not only a solitary pursuit, it is uniquely all-encompassing. Besides, for me the rudiments of ki had come through the tension of a bow, and I supposed that my improvement would be through further lessons in archery. The master, however, had other notions.

What he wanted me to do was find the arc of shooting a bow in all things, but first in my way of walking. The arc of the arrow becomes a metaphor to suggest the way to finding the ki potential in each activity. It stems from the esthetic poise of an archer and from the beauty of flight in a well shot arrow; that is, man transformed into an action. My teacher wanted me to transform, to keep my weight on my heels by lowering my center of gravity into my belly. He said that if I slowed down my breath, I would increase the ki by finding the rhythm in my steps. Speed didn't matter, as long as my breath moved my body correctly and concentrated my attention.

He said that with every breath we are standing between cosmos and self. What we don't always realize is how the self's rambling thoughts block out the distribution of ki, or how the constant rambling causes lapses of attention. After a while, it dawned on me that what he intended to teach me was quite specific: when to distribute what and where in the motions basic to walking or riding a horse so that I wouldn't block out the ki field. By not blocking the ki, he believed I would automatically get a grip on my thoughts. I would have to learn to work the rhythms of motion into a directed pattern that would become habitual. It was going to be a matter of endless repetition with an archetypal form called the Diamond Being or the Diamond Man. Using the diamond as an image for the form would come to have many ramifications as time went on, because this Diamond Being was the presence in mind I needed to develop. It is the archetype normally missing in the contemporary Western mind. Even its very existence is controversial.

In the beginning, the master didn't seem to want to talk to me about anything other than the way I was walking. I became rather self-conscious about my footsteps. He just smiled and suggested that I keep my torso still and take shorter steps, with feet farther apart and knees pointed outward. He gave me the assignment of walking around the stone house in my bare feet until the rhythm of breathing and walking became one without my thinking about it. I surmised that he didn't feel I could shoot my bow correctly until I became accustomed to the methodical pace. I kept looking for an opening to induce him to shoot his bow, so that I could shoot mine. Unfailingly, he avoided such a shooting match.

After catching me walking stoically around the house several mornings in a row, he gave in partially. He may have thought I'd never get my center of gravity low enough to please him.

"Walk as if you were shooting a bow," he suggested.

I walked around the stone house holding my bow at half-draw in front of me, like a hunter. I walked under the duress of the string's tension. I could just as well have been walking around carrying a heavy object. After some time the force of my footsteps and the pull of the string reached an equilibrium—I had invented a kind of balance. He commented only on the fact that I wasn't so short of breath anymore. He just grinned, looked down, and blew his breath out for what seemed the longest time imaginable. Then he demonstrated walking in league with gravity while blowing out the breath and taking short simple steps.

I made the altitude an excuse for not duplicating his long-winded pace. He said I would acclimate myself in due time. Again and again I went around the house stalking an invisible quarry. With each circuit the pull of the string forced me to lower my center of gravity to keep my balance. I became focused on finding a more comfortable way to proceed. Sure enough, the stance for holding the

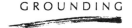

bow was causing me to lower my center of attention and increase my wind. I was working it out, solving the problem, but I wished I could do so by using the ki stored in my Diamond Being rather than my rapidly tiring muscles.

At night, as I tried to sleep through the muscle cramps in my upper back, I fought the long battle of impatience. The master spent most of his time in the woods, either walking or riding horseback. Often, there wasn't much else for me to do but visit with other people at the center; some of them were resident students of either archery or meditation, and others were seekers like myself. "Walk around in the woods with your bow as much as possible," the older students advised me. My one job seemed to be not to slip and fall. Even this was easier said than done. The ground was often treacherous—stones covered with pine needles—and the bow caught in branches or stuck in the ground when my attention was on the footing for the next step. The sought-for arc of ki that would map a way through the branches eluded me completely. Although I had watched the master's stride carefully, what he was doing remained a mystery.

As a teacher he was unlike any I'd known. The center ran on a haphazard schedule, without any strict requirements or regimens to follow. People came and went daily. We were each on our own, following suggestions made by the master but setting our own pace. We rarely spoke about religion, Buddhism or any other. The center might best be described as a complex of houses harboring people with an affinity for the master. He wandered around and, with one glance, seemed to know if it was advisable to speak with a student or to pass by. For him to be available, we had to be in some invisible harmony with him; to achieve this, a student or a visitor had to count on his own intuitive powers.

3

A   WALKING   LESSON

In American society we poke fun at those who move slowly, joking that someone can't walk and think at the same time. To improve ourselves we learn to tie many skills together, then we pride ourselves on the achievement. So it was quite a surprise when the master said I had to learn to walk and not think. "You have unknotting to do," he claimed.

The remarkable man who had shown me the point in my palm that stimulates the ki told me that the master spoke about unknotting from experience. When he first came to the States the master had discovered that students didn't automatically revere the teacher. The strict, traditional methods were not effective. He could teach only by winning people over, and to do this he had to rely on something other than language and personality. He could be effective only by following the simple way of self-containment. The more his students watched him in action, the more they were drawn to his style. I was told that even though he was an eminent historian of the traditions, he found himself teaching others by example rather than through discourse. He practiced the fundamentals of breath-posture and stance-attitude, as his spiritual ancestors had done to teach the Japanese aristocrats who were not Buddhists.

It was decided that I could best practice these basic principles by walking on the slope above the house. First, I studied the rudiments of the walking method by watching the master. For convenience, I have broken them down into four steps.

1. Keep knees and toes angled outward.
2. Take a half-stride forward with the left foot and place the heel down firmly.
3. Don't pivot onto the ball of the left foot before raising the right foot for a half-stride.
4. Place the weight onto the heel when landing.

In this heel-to-heel style of walking, the motion comes from swinging the leg from the hip socket rather than raising the knee. When done correctly, the torso seems to ride on the chariot of the legs. The essence of the step is a gliding balance that guides the motions.

I found that placing my heels firmly on the earth supported my body so that the weight was distributed along my spine. Keeping my feet spread apart on the ascent, I was able to move from side to side as I went up the incline. Since my weight remained under me at all times, my footing was secure. When it became harder to climb, I could still exhale and press out my belly while lowering my center of gravity by bending into the slope. The problem with this walking style was that I couldn't accelerate uphill, which disconcerted me. My pace was retarded by the side-stepping and by timing my breath, and it seemed as though it would take forever to go anywhere.

"What you lose in speed, you make up for in endurance," the master said. "I believe this is the lesson of your folktale about the tortoise and the hare."

It wasn't, but his mistake revealed a difference in perspective that was illuminating. Speed, which is a Western fascination, is irrelevant to grasping the arc of ki. He believed that by going slow, I would eventually discover the arc in the step, and the intuition of it would take me far beyond the moral of slow but steady. To aid me he picked up a four-foot-long branch, broke off the twigs, and suggested that it was a bow. I held the stick as I had held the bow when walking around the house. This forced me to balance my upper and lower body, and after a few minutes the difference was self-evident: I began to glide. It felt slow, yet the ground was moving quickly beneath me. He smiled at the instant I became aware of the distinction between moving with gravity and moving against it. My consciousness shifted even more than my sense of motion. In that moment, the colors of the valley and mountains stopped being colors I saw esthetically and became variations of intensity. I heard the difference between insects as they flew by. Truly, everything becomes visible when one begins to walk in a meditative state. The difference, other than speed, is the ability to discern the space that surrounds each step. The body moves in accord with the environment and yet independent of it. The more in accord, the lighter the step is; the more independent, the better the breathing is. It sounds mystical, but it really isn't. As the mind-body becomes an antenna for the world's flux, one sees both more and differently. The mind admits that it is a single corpuscle of blood drifting through a gigantic landscape of veins and arteries. The earth itself is the body for these veins, a realm of myriad greens, blues, browns, and yellows. I was convinced that the master was someone who could teach me to use my entire being to adjust to the new contours and make them my everyday reality.

It is difficult for a Westerner to remove ego from success. The satisfaction of accomplishment can alter the natural reflexes, adding superfluous motions and thoughts. What the master required was not self-satisfaction but self-containment. The specific advantage of his walking method was that it kept the torso steady so that the breathing remained constant, as if one were meditating. The general advantage was an increase of the sixth-sense faculty.

"Don't exhale until the tension shifts into the belly," the master warned. He stuck his thumb hard into the flesh just below his navel and let it bounce off a few times. "Balance goes down, then shifts up," he intoned, nodding in agreement with himself.

Not knowing exactly what he meant, I had to guess. If my guess was wrong, he'd correct me. Forcing me to guess and watch rather than explaining was itself an important part of his method. I was being forced to improve my intuitive power by organizing bodily movements and guesses into a pattern. I didn't have it right until the Diamond Being became a tangible presence in mind.

Through reminding myself that I was an integrated mind-body, a many-sided diamond rather than an abstracted personality, I could control my breathing and thus my inner reactions to thoughts. I could actually walk without daydreaming, my mind absorbed within the Diamond Being, letting the twinges of sensation flow through the mind-body prism. That is, I could sense enough of the arc of ki in my motions so that all thoughts were subjugated to its marvelous feel. The arc is, or rather contains, the waves and undulations that determine the "when" of the next step. The feeling is like waiting for waves to recede before stepping into the ocean. By recognizing the subtle feeling of the timing, the intuition guides the walker so that he or she doesn't separate mind and body. The results are evident in the attitude and appearance of the walker. While the feel of the Diamond Man is somewhat nebulous at first, practice with the steps of walking—like learning to walk all over again—allows the attention to become subtle and disciplined enough to discover this inner reality and its relationship to gravity.

By instinct we have a desire for fluidity. While walking with the master I became more fully aware of the correlation between fluidity and an easy self-containment. I relaxed as he surrounded me with the ease of his very practiced presence. Before my new awareness had any verbal dimension, he had me walking downhill rapidly while bracing myself with the center of gravity in my belly. Correct stance required keeping my head level even though my eyes looked down at the trail. Side-stepping made keeping my head back easier, and crouching kept the lowest point of the diamond, the coccyx, from wobbling. In effect, I was walking like an animal, and this is when the Diamond Man began to emerge from my original nature. It was as if the master, by running alongside me, had revealed the obvious.

For most of my life I'd assumed that the control of my actions depended on will power, fortitude, and intention. That it should depend on an ability to feel actions in a fluid flow of motion was sometimes evident when I had had a hotshot kind of day, but I'd never thought I could discipline myself to have the "feel" every day. Before I met my teacher I had only the vaguest clues as to the form of the innermost self where the sense of ki is stored. I was trying to digest the fact that there were schools of learning that didn't leave to chance the discoveries I needed to make.

4

THE DIAMOND BEING

I always listened when the master talked about concentrating the mind on the Diamond Being, but I felt cornered. I imagined sitting cross-legged and staring at a blank wall while my mind was forced to concentrate on a diamond image—or worse, to concentrate on emptiness. Meditation wasn't my cup of tea; I was even suspicious of the meditative look some people develop—that faraway gaze. Two of the younger students living with the master had this look, although with the master, who often drifted off, it was hard to be critical.

The subject of sitting in meditation had arisen when I complimented him on the cistern he'd built outside my cabin. Colored river stones were embedded in mortar, yet at first glance this rain barrel seemed overly decorative for the function. After a thundershower passed down the mountain, I was drawn to a closer examination of the cistern because the rain had increased the brightness of the stones. I saw that each had been placed in a geometric relationship to the others to form ribbons of matching color. The colors varied—ruby, green, grey, brown, quartz— as each stone became a piece of a larger jigsaw puzzle. Obviously, an enormous amount of attention had gone into their placement.

"But, no," he said. "I worked very fast, one stone right after the other." I didn't quite believe him—he had too wide a grin on his face. "But I scrutinized the pile of stones for quite a few hours before I placed them."

I gathered the stones left over from building the cistern with the intention of arranging them so that each one balanced against the curves or points of the adjacent ones. I stared intently at the thirty or so stones before moving them. I arranged shapes and colors in my mind quite easily, but when it came to moving them about with my hands I had to deliberate on each one. I tried to rush the deliberation and work quickly. The result was a terrible hodgepodge.

The master nearly laughed at my efforts. He hadn't meditated on the arrangement of the stones at all; rather, he'd meditated to enhance the skill of moving the mind quickly from point to point. When he was ready to place the stones, his mind was as nimble as his fingers. I asked for a description of the technique he used to keep his mind moving from point to point. He described the method, then sent me up the mountain to try it.

I sat on a rock outcrop above a ravine with the panorama of the valley before me. The steep chasm in front of me engendered the sensation of floating on a cloud. This spot had been recommended by the master, who had a knack for tailoring an exercise to a person's character. On the boulders it was relatively easy to do the type of sitting he required, and I relaxed.

I sat with eyes open but ignored the view, focusing on my own body or, at least, on points of it. In his method of mind-movement the master uses the ten points that delineate a diamond shape. The particular shape he has in mind looks like this:

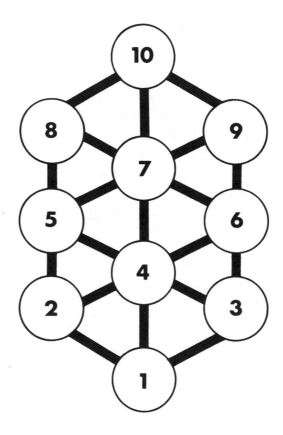

I drew imaginary lines from my groin up my sides to my head, then I drew a central column downward through the heart and navel to the groin. He had explained that to learn when to breathe and when to move in accord with the arc of ki, I needed some points of reference. Body terms were too imprecise for what he had in mind. Ten unmistakable pressure points, whose sensitivity to finger pressure are universal, provide an unambiguous map, and the diamond layout facilitates locating them. I wasn't sure where the points were until he pressed each one with a finger. First, one learns to find them with the fingers, then by recalling the pressure with consciousness alone.

It is best to locate the points in consciousness while sitting with legs crossed in front of you. The master said that I shouldn't sit with my weight jammed down through the sensitive point above the coccyx. Instead, the special point three fingers-width below the navel, which he calls the tanden, should come forward, and the two tender pressure spots in the hip joints should be drawn back. The net result of following his instructions was that my weight splayed to the sides as if I were sitting on a saddle. I was doing more than just sitting: I was contained in my sitting because the position emphasized—if not created—the Diamond Being.

"If you let the mind get stuck on one of the ten pressure points, both mind and point become very heavy and your body becomes like a corpse; you lose the life force," he said.

I never expected it to be so difficult to keep the mind moving. The master's last instruction was to concentrate on the ten points until my body disappeared and I, or "selfness," was contained wholly within the Diamond Being.

I sat on the rock with sunlight flickering through the spectral facets. It was a lovely image to hold onto; I could just lift off the rock and fly across the valley, a being of pure light and crystal. I could also become seriously deranged. If I wanted to accomplish the nearly impossible task of aiming a bow from a moving horse, however, I needed to become more accustomed to "flying."

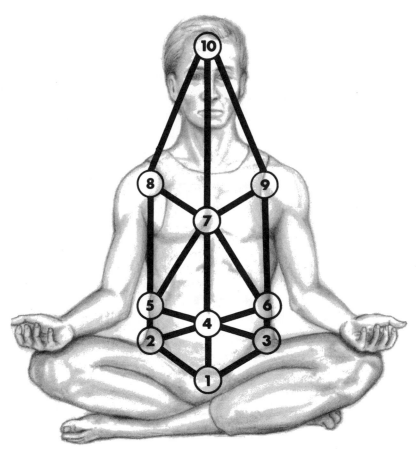

The diamond shape superimposes on the body to correlate specifically to ten pressure points. These ten points are the major centers of the ki that, together, determine the reality of the Diamond Being.

Dreaming about it wasn't the answer. I had work to do. There are many ways to move the attention from point to point. Starting at the top, I worked my way down the left side. Once at the groin I had to choose between going up my central column or up my right side. Stopping to decide, I learned what he meant about getting stuck at a point. To prevent the necessity of choice, I hit upon a pattern of criss-crossing from point to point. It worked once or twice, but the more involved I became, the more I had to check my memory to locate the next point. Again I was stuck, turning heavy. Given so many levels of specificity, thoughts about the body tangle the mind into a hapless switch-board. It was easier to tap the points with my finger than to think them. I let my finger do my thinking, then soon realized that in some inexplicable way it was distracting me from accomplishing my purpose.

I discarded this option and gazed off at the mountains across the valley. This calmed my mind, and I became more alert. I was impressed with the necessity of knowing when to stop doing something and change to another tack. At each insight into improving, the how-to of it became self-evident. Before, all options had seemed equal in value, and it was hard to know what to try. Not knowing what to do, I felt more inconsequential measured against these distances. Contrary to expectations, not knowing was helpful because I was able to realize that my true being was not best defined by anatomical description: it was more like a transparency composed of points that I could feel under-lying my body's form. I concentrated on these ten points so long and hard that they physically began to pulse. It was a task not only of meditating on a diamond image but of

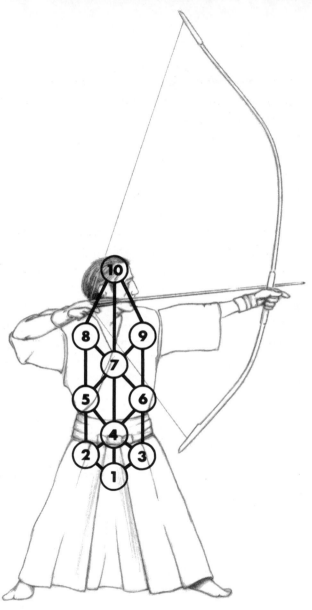

The mechanical lines of force located by the Zen archer travel through the ten points of the Diamond Being. These lines of force equate with the ki channels, as though archery taught man to locate the ki.

constructing one inside myself and then feeling the ki pass through its structure.

In a flash of insight I compared balancing my footsteps against the draw of a heavy bow with placing river stones in a pattern. My mind underwent a slow, steady set of adjustments through internal feedback until—despite all my premonitions of failure—I drifted into a feeling for the pattern. Once I felt it, the intuitive processes awakened. If I stopped to think about the next rock, the next step, or the next shot, some confusion was inevitable.

When I thought about sitting lightly on the rock, I became heavier, but when I kept my mind nimble the ki pulsed through the Diamond. Until I had freed myself of the bodily tensions no improvement took place. Of course, I had freed myself by breathing in the correct belly-out posture, my stance-attitude stimulated by the view. I dared to suppose that sitting in meditation while moving the mind through the points was what gave the master his buoyancy, and that there would come a time, after much practice, when my body image would change altogether, freeing me from old encumbrances.

I looked at my watch and saw that somehow three hours had gone by. Meditation had been far less boring than I'd expected. "You must learn to sit inside the drawn bow," the master had advised me. It was a puzzling statement. I had worked it over in my mind, deciding that he was drawing an analogy between the drawn bow's shape and the diamond form. Although the similarity did exist, he meant something more concrete, which wouldn't become apparent until I was sitting on a horse and nothing else other than the act of sitting on the horse existed.

"Not you but your Diamond Being sits on the horse and shoots," he had said. "Otherwise, you make the horse stumble."

Clearly, shooting a Zen arrow was not going to be a straightforward athletic exercise.

5

BREATHING HABITS

The master invited me to ride his horse. Looking forward to learning more about his skills, I put on riding boots and met him on the road. Along the horizon the sky was turquoise; above, it was dark blue. Small white clouds purified the greens of the field and trees. He wore baggy pants, a shirt, a bandana, and boots. We went to a shady spot where the grass was long and waited for his horse to stop grazing. In the meantime, he introduced the preparation for a riding meditation; in his world one had to prepare for a horseback ride just as a professor prepared for a lecture. He insisted that breathing exercises best tune the mind to the task at hand.

I was a bit nervous about riding a strange horse, and I hoped that the breathing exercises would calm my anxiety. The breathing rhythm depended on the type of person I was. To determine the most natural breathing pace for me, at his direction I jumped up and down in place for three minutes, paying attention to how many breaths I took. I was a two-medium-breath man, a completely different style from those who take three short, shallow breaths or one long, deep breath, as the master did. My rhythm was set to two medium-breath cycles, each lasting about twenty seconds, three in a minute. This was determined by the fact that I could exhale for about seventeen seconds.

Since I was having trouble with the duration of my breathing, the master suggested I place my index finger on my spine at the height of the hip bones. He said, "Breathe your three inhalations a minute for five minutes. Imagine a pool of water forming where the finger rests. Sustaining focus, you begin to heat this pool of water. When the pool becomes warm, a stream flows to the hips. This will strengthen the base that rests on the saddle and will increase the circulation around the navel and heart."

Okay, I thought, more circulation means more oxygen in the bloodstream, which will allow me to inhale less frequently. I spent five minutes squatting and breathing until the altitude seemed irrelevant. I was amused that I looked something like a baseball catcher waiting in a crouch. What I was waiting for, though, was not a pitch but for an expansion of the belly. Too flat a belly shows the teacher that the student isn't drawing up the breath from the lowest area and that the spine is too relaxed. When the four points at the base of the diamond aren't properly aligned, the ki cannot reach the upper torso. He knew what was going on because he watched my muscles during each breath.

His main advice was to correlate my breathing pattern with the stance that we called the powershift. The position was so named for two reasons. First, attention shifts from what goes on inside the head to what goes on in the belly. Second, strength shifts from the muscular plane to the psycho-physical plane. The stance depends on how the ten points of the diamond are accentuated by the position of the muscles and skeleton. Each movement is meant to aid the curvature of the spine and the bracing of the tanden.

The powershift developed during the period when the nobility hunted and fought with bows from horseback. They found the spine curved in at the lower back to be the most reliable position on the saddle—the same posture used today in dressage. The idea is that, when assuming this posture favorable to deep belly breathing, the rider is in the best position to shoot an arrow accurately.

I put a blanket and saddle on the small Indian Paint, adjusted the stirrups, and mounted. We needed no bit or reins for the lesson, just a halter and lead.

"Drop your shoulders and let your belly relax as you inhale," the master demanded. I took a medium breath through my nose, relaxing my abdomen. "Next, blow breath slowly through your lips and push your abdominal muscles outward as you exhale so that it feels like you are breathing out against your navel."

Because I was in a saddle it was actually easier to blow my breath out by rolling my abdominal muscles downward rather than by collapsing my chest. I found that an exhale controlled by squeezing the muscles that pushed at the navel was steady and even. Also, the breath seemed to last longer. Of course, this was a most unnatural feeling. In the past it had never occurred to me to press my belly out by pressing down with my shoulders as I exhaled.

"The movement is correct when you feel a down-turning crescent under your rib cage," the master said. "It may take several tries to form this crescent. As soon as you have done so, pull in the small of your back, increasing the natural indent. Your posture will come undone if you inhale and fail to slide your hip joints back into the rise of the saddle. Exhale and push the breath hard against the navel until it knots there. Better straighten your head until the spine holds it, then bring your toes up and your heels down, or else you will fall off."

The threat of falling made me listen, since I had no bit or hackamore. I focused both my attention and breath in my lower abdomen. As the horse moved, I felt a coiled spring's tension inside me. I was solidly anchored, and the horse acted as if it were accustomed to my posture even though I had never been on it before. The faster the stride, the more I leaned forward and relaxed my weight into the saddle.

I had just become comfortable when the master suddenly clapped his hands once, loudly. The horse bucked in surprise, and I certainly would have fallen if the spring weren't coiled through me. Where did this compressed energy of balance come from, and how was it induced by a change of posture? Before the master had combined the breathing technique with the powershift such inner balance seemed totally implausible. Afterward, it was self-evident, and I understood why the ki must be distributed through the ten points of the Diamond Being. It boils down to this: the indwelling force of the ki can accentuate the elasticity of the channels between the points; this balances and strengthens the body's infrastructure. Using this principle, elderly chi masters in China can hold a rope against ten younger men.

Any flaws in the ten-point diamond stance that impede the breath are obvious to the master. If the powershift (illustrated on pages 48–54) is not combined with the timing of the breath, the power of the ki cannot be tapped. A student quickly learns the two main lessons: (1) the breath-posture, which combines the breathing pattern with the outward-pressed belly, and (2) the stance-attitude, which focuses the subconscious mind into myriad internal adjustments that free the mind-body from the external tension that blocks the ki. The two lessons are interdependent, and one cannot transcend the failure to master either.

For a Westerner the major problem is always the emphasis on breathing, and an incorrect posture that impedes slow, steady breath. Correct breathing keeps the mind calm as difficulty and exertion increase. It keeps the meditative pace of slow motion centered in the squeezing of the abdominal muscles. When air is released through the mouth at a slow, constant rate, inhaling becomes automatic. At the end of the breath, the belly is almost flat, except for the navel area. On the inhale, the lower abdomen drops as if a girdle had been removed from it. This is the girdle of mental tension that retards the body's elasticity.

The master noticed how much more rapidly I inhaled when the horse trotted. Because of it, I could not exhale for seventeen seconds. I inhaled too frequently, and he emphasized that the body is most vulnerable during inhalation. I was not to let the motion of the horse change my breathing rhythm, because it would soon alter my stance-attitude. I would lose all sense of the arc of ki, which I needed to align with to be a competent horse archer.

To align with the arc—the pattern in the flux—I had to use my breathing as a timing device. The master had me pretend to hold a bow and aim at a bale of straw in the pasture. If I timed my breath right, I would pass the bale just as the exhale was about to end. The pattern always emerges more clearly near the end of the breath. The pattern is the same thing as an intuitive feeling.

The ancient masters had two problems to solve. The first was the problem of the horse's up-and-down motion, which caused the view of the target to bounce. The second was lining up the arrow with the target while moving laterally, which produced relativity distortions. Long before Einstein's theory of relativity, the masters had to deal with the type of illusion that occurs when horses cross in opposite directions. To solve these two problems required transforming the way in which the intuitive senses worked. To resolve the problem of speed and position, the archer needed to "see" in slow motion; to solve the vertical bouncing of the target, the archer had to locate an apex in the trajectory incalculable by normal means. Both time and space had to be grasped in a new way. No wonder a special school or tradition had to be sustained, a school with techniques different from those used to train stationary archers. No wonder the traditions of this school baffled the imagination and evoked the world of mystical powers. The practice of Zen had nothing to do with magic, however, and everything to do with posture, stance, and what the masters called the "original nature." Animals in their natural state could move through space and time without being overcome by illusions. The masters taught humans to reclaim the same natural ability.

I discovered that as I increased the time between my inhales to seventeen seconds and pressed the breath against the belly as I blew air through my mouth, my ability to feel the arc of ki and to see in slow motion increased. As long as I kept my spine indented and my heels lowered as I posted up and down, my body remained a spring. It uncoiled for an instant as I rose, coiling up again as I came down. If I inhaled only at the second before rising, I was more stable and more in harmony with the horse.

It wasn't until I got off the horse that I could recap what I'd done and practice breathing on the ground. From riding correctly, I had gathered the feel of the breathing that best augmented the powershift. It was the opposite of what I had always done. All my life I'd inhaled for strength, but now I had to change my habit and inhale for repose.

6

THE BODY AS BOW

I don't want the ki to sound esoteric and out of reach. Holding your arms in front of you, direct your palms down at a forty-five-degree angle, pressing your ring finger into your palm. From that point of contact you can imagine a line to the ground. You can also intuitively feel a beam—or arc—from your palm to the ground if you set yourself in the ten-point stance and press your attention along the arc. The arc comes out of your palm as you push your breath against the tanden. The imagined line and the intuited line are qualitatively different: the former exists only as a wish, the latter supports your entire body. One is just mind, the other is a combination—the mind-body.

Since making a claim like this may be baffling, I suggest that we look at the arc of ki from the perspective of organization. Following a sequence according to the changes at each stage turns chaos into order, imagination into intuition. What I believe I do to attain the ki is to organize my mind-body on a more subtle, complex level of order than usual. It was the master who required me to do this, and archery that reinforced the sequence. Yet this ordering of the mind-body into the Diamond Being can be done without either the master or the bow, without a teacher and without an external aid. It requires only the solitary work of practicing until the arc of ki braces the palms while the student leans the mind-body in one direction or the other.

In this solitary work it is impossible to judge progress from the reactions of others. In fact, most of us are so thoroughly habituated to competition that in its absence we can't tell whether or not we are increasing our awareness. Nor can we determine if we have discovered the ki from objective results such as hitting the bull's-eye. Discovery of ki is a subjective accomplishment, an intuition of harmony. The bio-chemical feeling of the body's electrical energy isn't enough; in fact, it may be irrelevant. There are instructors who can teach you to feel this electricity or how to hit the target every time. There are also masters who can instruct you in the development of the ki. The two kinds of teachers and their two very different kinds of instruction should never be confused. And although the ki masters often owe their allegiance to Eastern traditions, the East does not have an exclusive claim to this knowledge; many cultures have used similar methods to increase the sense of the field of life. It is very nearly a telepathic ability.

If the master sees that a student is losing interest because of an inability to find the arc that unites his or her actions with the outside world, he may decide to transmit a few pointers. It is equally likely that he will decide that the student's floundering will increase the effort of concentration. The master's tremendous patience is part of his overall serenity. He isn't a shaman with a wonderful bag of tricks, he is an example—the exemplar. He acts as if he were the only human being on the planet, self-contained; and this, oddly, is why he is so available to those who need him. In his world, what is absolutely essential is that he is not self-absorbed; thus, he can react openly and clearly to any person or situation. His mind-body work is psychic.

The teachers say that if you arrange your body into the ten-point lattice of the Diamond Being and breathe rhythmically from the belly, many ki phenomena will occur, leading to knowledge of the cosmos and the self. Although the Diamond can be taught in various ways, using different primary patterns, the resulting "feel" is universal. An interested reader may ask, "In what pattern did he arrange his points to attain this feeling of the ki?" and, "What can I do?" The caveat is that this "doing" takes years rather than months to perfect. Still, many changes occur in the early experimenting; the breath capacity increases steadily, for instance.

To demonstrate what I do when I enter the Diamond Being, I will present a sequence and describe what occurs when I go through it. The object of the sequence is to turn the body into a bow. This may sound strange but it is possible to make the body store the ki like a bow stores the energy for sending an arrow. The master sees the spine as an inner bow that can be strung by sequentially moving the muscles to create the bowed posture and by breathing in relationship with these movements. He is, of course, thinking of a Japanese-style bow (see page 75). I think of this recurved bow as an instrument that borrows time from gravity by projecting the arrow, and I think of the mind-body as an instrument that stores gravity as energy for the moment of release. Before I learned the powershift my body fought with gravity; afterward I felt lighter on my feet, as though I was becoming weightless to some extent. Balance and the pull of gravity become real concerns when riding a galloping horse while holding and aiming a bow with both hands. The rider must be as light as possible.

The powershift sequence begins with a separation of my attention from the surroundings. I ignore who is around me and where I am. There are people and places that generate a nervous tension which is difficult to overcome, yet success depends on ignoring them. The first instruction is to relax inward and combine posture and breath so that the belly becomes the center of the universe. In other words, the first step in the sequence is to draw the mental attention into the tanden. This is done by imaging the body as the staff of a short bow with the handle being just below the navel. The stringing of the bow (the spine) begins in the first movement of the sequence by standing up straight and letting the belly protrude forward like the bow handle. The feet are close together and the spine indents slightly with the weight of the body on the toes. I inhale deeply and let out a sigh of relief that I can slouch, then inhale deeply once more.

The second step takes me to the first point of the Diamond Being, the groin, as I draw the coccyx back. To make this easier, I spread my feet wide and shift my weight to my heels. This step automatically indents the lower spine and puts some more pressure on the abdominal muscles that surround the tanden. It's like attaching a string at the lowest tip of the spine and pulling it upward. The lower tip of a recurve bow will bend back as the bow is strung. I exhale slowly as the tailbone slides back.

The third step is to move the hips, points two and three, first down and forward, then up and back. Going forward requires bending the knees and going up and back requires straightening them. This rotation locks the lower spine into the indented position, drawing the coccyx back as far as possible. When sitting in meditation, the same adjustment takes the weight off the tailbone and disperses it into the buttocks. In the standing position this hip excursion leaves the spine more flexed, or bowed, allowing me the freedom to really expand my belly and breathe against the tanden point. During the third step, I concentrate on the long exhale.

Now I tense the two side points, five and six, and bend backward from them, as if someone were drawing a bow and forcing the upper limb of the spine as far back as the lower one. I am aware of bending only as far back as needed to bring my head and shoulders into the same plane as my buttocks. This movement bows the body as if there was an invisible string between the back of the head and the coccyx. The top abdominal muscles form a muscular crescent under the rib cage. As I continue to exhale after bending back, there comes a conscious feeling of my heartbeat. The shortness of breath is coupled with an increased awareness of my blood pumping. At this time I become self-centered in the best sense of the word: I am inside myself, and the attention that usually resides in the eyes and mind drops completely into the body.

In the fifth step of the sequence I continue the backward bend of the upper body by lifting my shoulders and rotating them back. The belly really juts forward now and my exhaling breath seems to be pumping it up. Both limbs of the bowed spine are back as far as they can go; however, I am out of balance, immobilized by this awkward bending that strains the lower back. It takes a long time to get accustomed to the strain; after a while a set of muscles emerge in this area at the small of the back and the spine becomes more flexible here. There is also considerable tension under the clavicle, points eight and nine. The arms feel lighter, like wings. I bend my knees for balance.

The sixth step is meant to adjust and compensate for the tensed, bowed position. Without changing the backward-bending posture, I tilt my skull forward and let the weight of the head shift my body weight forward a bit. As the abdominal muscles knot at the tanden, (a very subtle sensation), the shoulders which were rotated back shift down without coming forward. This downward thrust of the shoulders presses out the tanden to its fullest possible extension. The body is at full draw, so to speak, the action of pressing the rotated shoulders down increasing the curve in the upper back to its fullest extent. I am aware of the arc of ki reaching from my tailbone to my cranium. Leaning slightly forward while remaining locked in the drawn-bow position eases the tension of storing so much ki, or so much energy, in the mind-body. (In employing the powershift while shooting a bow from horseback, I actually start pulling the string using the expanded abdominal muscles to hold the bow's tension at the tanden. To lean back instead of forward would cause me to lose both momemtum and balance on the saddle.) The knees are bent as if one were ready to jump outward.

Near the very end of the exhale, I proceed to the

seventh and final step of the powershift. Slowly lifting my head upright and allowing my spine to follow, I align the tenth point of the Diamond Body by letting my skull wander around until I feel it balance on the tip of my spine—now my eyes are level enough to direct an arrow or a shout. In the mirror I appear to be standing naturally, but I feel the tension of being drawn back as if someone behind me were pulling the invisible string between the back of my head and my tailbone. I feel the lines of force moving through the points of the Diamond Being. These lines are felt as muscular tensions, pulsations, and circuits of bio-chemical electricity.

Ancient teachers became aware that archery training altered the mind-body. They knew that the weapon, the bow, and the man became one indistinguishable unit. They knew that becoming aware of the arc of ki in the spine was as physical an experience as becoming aware of the tension in a bow when handling it. With the ki stored in the mind-body, the archer becomes free to act in the eternity of the moment. A mental picture of his Diamond Being fills the cavities of his mind, and the image of the self as a solid vanishes into the greater realities of energy and flux. My teacher says the mind is like a crystal wherein the thoughts create the lattice of reality. It is an intricately woven fabric—mind and reality. My experiences begin to suggest that there is nothing that isn't the mind's extension and that those patterns which are most clear are the ones which mesh with or invoke the ki. Sages have always asserted that this mesh comes from a concentration focused inward and they mean this literally, physically, and then by extension, psychologically. Although this looking inward is a very old teaching, the reasons for doing it need restating in a new vocabulary for each generation so that they can be transmitted from age to age without sounding farfetched.

The act of looking inward can mistakenly be taken as an exercise in thought. But, in every sense, thinking or writing about looking inward is an act of translation, from one culture and generation to another, and from one manner of articulation to another. The same mental powers that adjust words on the page adjust muscles and points of the mind-body: writing or thinking alone does not bring the fullest intuitive power into play. Looking inward means experiencing the powershift and eventually discovering the Diamond Being, the truest inner self. Paradoxically, this self is not very individualistic; rather, it is the self we most share in common. The intuitive self is actually telepathic with the world and others. Alive and aware within the Diamond Body, it is possible to look at the stars and feel their energy coursing within.

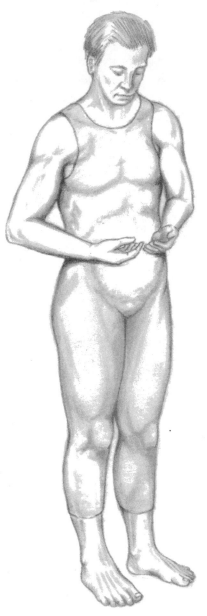

1. The powershift is a standing meditation that provides all the benefits of sitting meditation yet allows these benefits to be transferred to any action. The first position is relaxation, a sigh of relief as one looks down at the ground and allows the belly to absorb the weight of the chest and shoulders. Let the belly protrude forward. Arms are bent at the elbow and the hands are held palms up at the level of the navel. The student inhales through the nose with an attitude of attention, letting the body's weight fall all the way to the ankles, shoulders leaning forward. With the inhale the student becomes aware of the importance of air to the biological self, breath to the organization of movement, and breathing to the openness of mind. The inhale teaches humility.

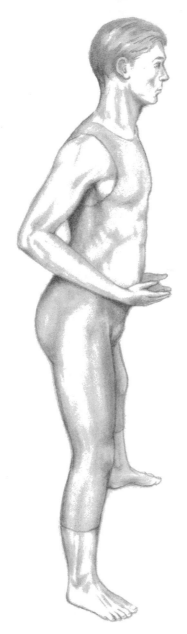

2. The second position counters the over-relaxation of the first. The start of the exhale is accompanied by an expansion of the abdominal muscles. The head is raised to plumb and the feet are spread apart almost as far as they will go so that the body looks like an hourglass. The student must be fully embracing gravity before he can achieve the main movement of the second step, that is to slide the coccyx back without pulling the belly in, keeping the weight of the body over the heels. The elbows are drawn back slightly to aid in this movement. Concentrate on the open palms to remind yourself that mind and body are not separate, then close the fingers into the hand.

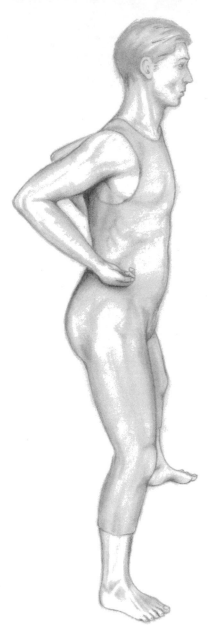

3. The third step still concentrates on moving the tip of the spine back, thereby almost raising the buttocks. The hips are slid down and then hiked back; they are rotated in this way so that the tailbone can be locked into its pushed-back position. This hip movement also allows the lower belly to sink into the groin, thereby making it more convex. Exhaling slowly, think of blowing up a baloon that resides in two places: outside the lips and within the belly. The effort of blowing air out the mouth regulates the expansion of the abdominals. It takes a slow steady pressure. The student feels an expansion of potential as the burden of the mind controlling the body is shifted to the tanden. "I am becoming a bow," I tell myself. Find the spot in the palm that is sensitive to the fourth finger and feel the lines of force, the sinews of ki.

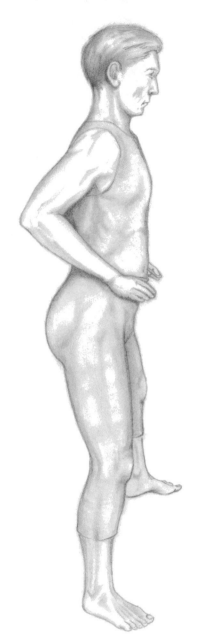

4. To begin the fourth step, pull the elbows all the way back and up, and then bend backward from points five and six of the Diamond Being until the shoulders and upper back are in the same plane as the buttocks. Extend through the cervical spine by seeking the sky with your vision, keeping the nose and chin as level as possible. The wrists are level with the navel, fingers reaching downward to the hipbones.

Bending back from here pushes the belly out—the protruding belly is the center of gravity, the handle of the bow. This full extension of the spine causes the muscles of the chest to lengthen around the heart and the blood to pump through the heart at a much-quickened rate due to the duration of the exhale. The belly is half full and the lungs are half empty. This extreme position makes one aware of the ten points of the Diamond Being. You feel very powerful and alert, as if all the strings in the body were wound tight.

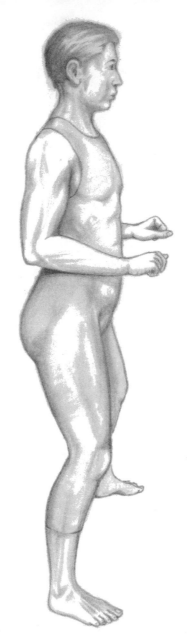

5. *The fifth step is to fully bow the upper limb of the spine. To do this the shoulders are lifted and rolled back. The chin is tucked in while the head remains back. At this stage, the body is fully braced, the bow is strung. The thumbs are brought forward to the end of the protruding belly and the fourth fingers are now driven into the palm so that the finger activates the nerve ending. The magnetic twinge runs all the way to the shoulders, through points eight and nine.*

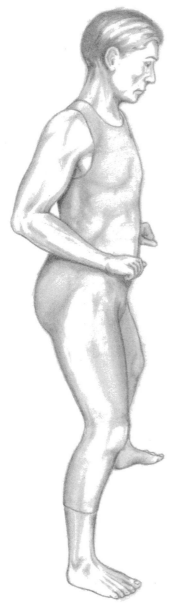

6. If the bow is not to break—if the ki is to flow—the stressed body must become more flexible. Bend the knees, allowing the weight of the head to shift the body weight slightly forward. The spine, from the tailbone to the point between the shoulders, remains in the bowed position. Press the shoulders down and curve them forward, sending two lines of force to empty the lungs and so extend the tanden to its fullest outward capacity. Pressing the shoulders down locks the bowed curvature into the upper spine, which prevents losing the stance when one leans forward over the center of gravity at the tanden. The weight remains on the heels even when leaning forward. To assist in maintaining balance while leaning forward, slide the arms forward and project a line of force downward from the pressure point on the center of your palm, or imagine that you have a ski pole in each hand from which you are pressing yourself away from the ground. Leaning forward and bending the knees makes the whole body more supple; the rigidity developed by getting into the bowed position is eliminated. The position is set so you can really just relax all the muscles and let the body's weight fall forward. The curvature of the spine prevents you from tumbling over. Gravity is now working with, rather than against, the body weight. You feel lighter, irrepressible.

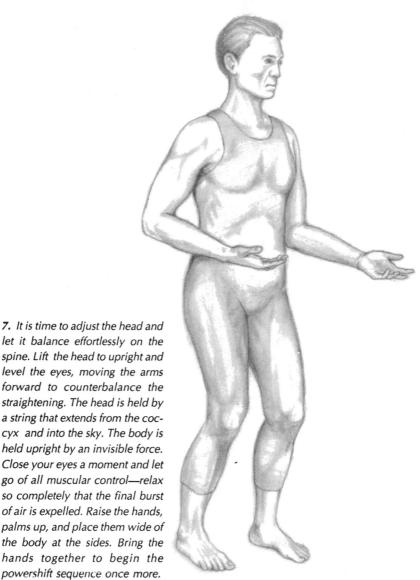

7. It is time to adjust the head and let it balance effortlessly on the spine. Lift the head to upright and level the eyes, moving the arms forward to counterbalance the straightening. The head is held by a string that extends from the coccyx and into the sky. The body is held upright by an invisible force. Close your eyes a moment and let go of all muscular control—relax so completely that the final burst of air is expelled. Raise the hands, palms up, and place them wide of the body at the sides. Bring the hands together to begin the powershift sequence once more.

Know that anything is possible now. The arrow may go through the target or squirt into the ground—it doesn't matter. You are not afraid to miss or make a mistake. You are the bow, filled with enormous energy, paradoxically stressed to the limit and yet completely flexible.

7

THE STANCE

In each week of practice my progress resembled a bouncing ball: I would improve and then regress, my self-assessment going up and down.

"You must turn your body inside out," the master said. I tried not to laugh at the image conjured up by his difficulty with English, for he was intensely serious. We stood on a flat boulder at the crest of the hill above the stone house. It had been a steep climb. Trees blocked out the valley, but the road dropped sharply below us. He seemed convinced that my attitude wasn't correct because my head wasn't balanced on my spine. I would never have connected this physical fact with my mental state, yet for him the correlation between stance and attitude was direct. The body either reveals the state of mind or influences it, I didn't know which.

"Don't watch me, watch my ten points" he advised, and demonstrated what he meant by the correct stance. I realized quickly enough how difficult it was to watch all his moves at once. It was necessary to feel the stance inside myself to understand what he was doing, which meant I had to have the right attitude. Attitude depends on self-containment, and I hadn't been well enough integrated, so

I'd been rather unsteady. Maybe the bouncing-ball effect explained why he taught correct attitude through the stability of the stance.

I watched him plant his feet wide apart, toes pointing out. By planting his feet, I mean he placed each foot down with all his weight firmly on the heel. He leaned over at a thirty-degree angle, staring at the rock surfaces below him. I wanted to reach out and catch him before he fell over the edge, but he never wavered. Keeping his arms on the outer edge of his torso, he put both arms out in front of him with the palms facing up. He bent his elbows slightly and drew them back toward his body. The arm motion caused his hips to slide back and his belly to bulge downward. He reminded me of a diver about to leap into the water.

From the powershift he went into his stance. He pulled his elbows back until his hands were even with his sides. He faced the ground and paused, gathered himself in some unfathomable way, then turned his palms over. His fingers hovered above his feet. It seemed an awkward position, with the coccyx bone and rear end curved upward. He had turned his hands over, lifted himself, and shoved his buttocks back an inch or two more than normal.

He drew his hands back to his sides, turned them over once again, this time curling his fingers into his palms. His ring finger was pressed hard into the center of his palm, and at the same time he drew his head back, eyes looking straight ahead. By pulling his chin in, he centered his head on his neck and spine. He sniffed the air and curled his lower lip, creating a square jaw. Last, he leaned foward, and at this point, I knew what was happening. This was a kind of dance routine he used to set himself into an attitude suited for total outer awareness and internal concentration.

His stance, hence his attitude, was a far cry from the military ideal of belly in, chest out, shoulders back with a stolid glance. He bent his knees and kept his chest flat and open; that is, his heart area wasn't compressed by the pectoral muscles. His abdomen bulged out and his shoulder blades rotated down to drive a line of force right through his heels. He was completely relaxed, under no tension or rigidity, a reed in the wind.

I had watched what he did, but I hadn't even dreamed his interpretation. He showed me that his upper body was bowed forward and braced at the tanden the way a tripod braces a camera. The third leg, he claimed, was an invisible arc going from the tanden point to the ground. The arc from the tanden was like the arc from the palm of the hand but ten times stronger.

I took one of his long arrows, braced its metal point against my tanden and the other end against the ground, and pushed against it with my abdominal muscles. The arrow braced me as if it were the front leg of a tripod. I removed the arrow, pushed my tanden out, and stood in the powershift. While breathing against my belly I discovered that in place of the arrow was an invisible line of ki going from my body to the ground. I could swear by the feeling of the arc of ki issuing from my body, because the line remained after I'd pulled the arrow away, and something held me back: it may have been a pulsation of ki.

The master said, "In order to study, your mind must be involved in every motion. This is how you will join mind and body into one unit. It's no mystery, the mind-body; it's the result of much work."

Why hadn't he told me this before? I would have watched the way he organized his movements into discrete parts he could concentrate his mind on. He was working with nuances I hadn't imagined. Once again I leaned forward in the kneeling position, faced the ground, then raised myself until my hands were joined straight over my head and my backside touched my heels. Although I did my best to straighten myself as slowly as possible, I moved twice as fast as he did. He could demonstrate and give lessons, but no matter what he said or did I didn't learn anything until my self-instruction process stopped and my innate senses guided my movements in a kind of slow motion. My intuitive sense of time and space was improving, becoming less stressed and thus more sensitive. The ki resides in the slowness of the means. It was obvious now. Setting the stance leads to the weightless solidity that I would come to associate with the way of self-containment, and this change in turn influences the student's attitude. I no longer thought of myself in the same way once I became more familiar with the Diamond Being; maybe this Being was my enlightened self? I don't think I was any smarter, but I was more aware of the life force, the Seiki, which rhymes, coincidentallly, with psyche.

To be set in the stance is to feel invincible and at the same time to realize that one is completely vulnerable and insignificant. Only in this seemingly paradoxical state can one reach the correct attitude for riding and shooting without any concern other than the arc of ki. What happens otherwise is trivial, for the arc of ki is much like the Tao, heaven's way.

8

ATTITUDE

The master says that self-absorption—being concerned primarily about what may or may not happen—stifles the original nature and prevents the ki from energizing the lower torso. And yet I can never quite ignore how steep a hillside is or how high above the ground I am when a horse trots across a field rutted by summer rains. If there are numerous flies and wasps around, my anxiety increases, leading to the self-absorption of the shallow breath. My head falls forward, my chest closes up, and my toes point down in the stirrup. I usually catch myself only after the danger has passed.

Even though tough situations require the most grace under pressure, invariably, the rougher the conditions are, the harder it is to concentrate on correct breathing and posture. This discrepancy between what we should do and what we do is exactly the reason for the master's teaching. He says that the opposite of what we do naturally in an emergency is what is truly natural. Others may get excited and panic, but we should be calm and centered. Our attention and alertness should remain focused, because we concentrate on abdominal breathing and the form of the Diamond Being.

The master's way is much easier to preach than to

practice. It would be wonderful if the powershift could be reserved for whenever I wanted to use it, but this is not how inner concentration arises. The powershift must be practiced until it becomes second nature. Riding a horse in rough terrain with the ever-present possibility of falling off is a practice that, like meditation, concentrates the powershift. From the minute I step onto the saddle I must remember the dressagelike breathing posture and the master's calm attitude. The little reminders that I am not concentrating are a stumbling gait, a flat belly, rounded shoulders, and rapid breaths—suddenly I am off balance. But if I reinitiate the powershift, breathing in and blowing out through both mouth and navel at a steady rate, then I start riding uphill with the horse rather than dragging it down. It is all a matter of attitude, a word that should have nothing to do with confidence.

"The first test of your training will come when you shoot the bow from your horse. The second test will be how you act afterward."

The proper attitude in the stance isn't a mystery: one is spiritually minded, which is to say, "I am doing this for the sake of my Diamond Being and all material concerns be damned."

Once, on the return from the pasture to the stone house, the teacher tested my attitude by passing in front of me with a pert little smile. He suddenly stopped, and the moment I walked by he went behind me, and I felt his presence attacking my ankles.

"How am I going to keep my composure with you on my tail?" I wanted to ask him.

The answer was simple: I must not focus on the master.

Focus on breathing as if I were alone in the woods. Stand as if I were shooting an arrow. Move as if I were on the horse. My attitude is wrong if I play the game. I had to ignore the master; a subtle lesson, indeed, for any student.

I knew he was using this playful technique to teach, and he knew that I understood. This made it even harder not to play the game.

"Knowing what to do and when is the result of a clear mind," he'd say. He believes that every thought and every anxiety produces a reaction in the gut that alters the breath-posture and hence the stance. Trying to clear the mind and stop reacting only causes more stress. A clear mind is empty of reactions, not of the thoughts that generate them. The minute I tell myself not to fall at the deep ditch, I subconsciously start to fall at that spot. I used to avoid this autosuggestive trap by thinking about something irrelevant to what I was doing. The trouble with this technique was that I lost the precision necessary to do the task flawlessly.

Riding a horse while trying to arrange the bow and arrow is like trying to walk normally while the master is stepping on your heels. Where do you put your attention first? The clear mind is in a selfless mode, reacting only to the breeze. Self-confidence quickly leads to self-absorption. There must be no master and no horse, just walking and riding.

Only if I kept checking each point on the Diamond, so that my mind moved freely and I was aware of each part of me, could I walk without stumbling. Even thoughts about how well the master timed his step to mine didn't unnerve me. He'd say that the clear mind is in the free association of intuition, meaning that the path is neither judgmental nor reactive and thus is clear. Intuition decides that calmness or anger is the best arrow for the moment, and intuition cannot become stuck on its last move.

Instead of taking the road for the last hundred yards, he skirted the edge, which was nothing but tire-tossed stones. I was now irrationally determined to show him I could keep my center of gravity in my belly on rocks, too. I bent my knees and took short, carefully placed, side-to-side steps. Sure enough, I kept pace with him, until he abruptly turned around and cut across my stride, smiling.

"You are doing just what you were doing wrong when you walked around the stone house holding your bow. I can hear too much time elapse between your steps. Your weight is overbearing your stride. I could knock you over by clapping my hands. If not me, the mountain will knock you off at any time."

He smiled because my mistakes were amusing. Of course he was correct; I was using my will power to follow him, not my internal buoyancy, my clear being. The master knows just when to intervene, as if he were psychic; he didn't criticize my attitude until I was least ready to admit the error of my ways. Only when I thought I was doing very well could I respond with enough attention to his revelation that I was cheating. Determination was making me heavy. A spiritual attitude is always light.

It takes immersion in the stance to know when it is best to try and do something. No matter how much ki resonance he put into the clap he threatened me with, the critical decision would be when to bring the hands together so that the clap would be effective. He couldn't

decide when to clap if he was reacting to my confusion—
I had to not-think, too.

I wondered why I had followed him onto the rocks. I could have walked abreast of him and stayed on the road. I had played the game, but now something prodded me to escape. I was suddenly listening to an inner voice, the voice he called intuition. This barely intelligible prompting came from—or resided in—the grinding of his feet on loose rocks. I was catching on. "Get back on the road," the voice said. Training the intuition meant becoming calm enough to hear the messages behind ordinary perceptions. Growing calm enough to have an unclouded attitude depends on making the adjustments of the stance, and this is why stance and attitude are, in this training, inseparable.

9

THE INNER PULSES

After a few more weeks of archery practice, I reached a new stage: the development of pulsations at the ten points of my Diamond.

All of us have experienced the throbbing sensation produced by a wound healing. This throbbing, or pulsing, is what I felt. The pulses would start in my heart and shift to the other points. Wherever I put my attention I drew on a different well. The master said these pulses were generated by the ten wells of ki, which are located at the pressure points. In a healthy person, the strength of the pulsations is equal at each well; illness causes weakness at the affected wells.

I had a fairly good idea of the relation between well points and body parts while under the tension of the bow. Entering deeply into the powershift through archery caused a momentary shortness of breath that forced my heart to pump faster. If I breathed within the posture for two or three cycles, my heartbeat returned to normal and the pulsations slowed down. At that point, I was set and concentrated, the purpose of the shift achieved. The heartbeat remained something I could call on, and, when I envisioned a ki well pulse, my heart pulse would increase. To direct my attention to one of the pulses, I blew my breath very slowly into a point, especially at the tanden.

In these pulses I had made a discovery of a curious nature, but I had no idea what use to put it to. Although I mused about the ordinary electric currents of the human body, they did not equate with the pulses. Electric currents are extreme in creatures like the firefly and the electric eel. Their bodies generate a visible, palpable charge, in one case to attract a mate, in the other to stun prey. The eel's charge is strong enough to hurt a human, but it is not the result of the abiding ki, since it is generated by muscular action. Ki cannot shock anyone because it isn't based on an electric charge of any voltage, weak or strong. It can be amplified, though, so that it will course through the mind-body in a way that, because of the structure of the human nervous system, seems to be an electric shock. No other science exists for the pulses, and some physics of the ki is sorely needed.

The master knew full well that I was the sort who wouldn't be happy without a theory; just feeling the pulses wasn't enough for me. Rather than assuage my needs and provide one, he came up with an exercise to improve my abilities, assuring me that if I practiced it as much as I drove a car, the results would be self-explanatory.

"You need to catch your breath" was the way he stated what I had to do.

I had been trying to get the two weakest pulses, felt in my sides, to be as strong as the others. He suggested that there was another procedure to develop the strength of the ki but it would sound illogical to me. The exercise he proposed was to lower the rate and strength of the pulses in order to raise them to new levels. He wanted me to take the throbbing and slowly, using both mental and physical means, diminish it by increments to a rate of quietude.

He put his finger to my forehead and instantly I felt a throbbing issue from his finger; obviously, he could direct the pulse into his hands. The impact of his directed attention caused my eyes to blink uncontrollably.

"You respond," he suggested, and I found it easy to raise the pulse in my forehead to the same level as the pulse in his finger. I must admit I was looking at him with a bit of amazement since he could do such things so unpretentiously. His touch was so soft and so respectful of my space that I had an inkling of the depths of inner stillness generating such a strong finger pulsation.

"Respond," he said again. My awareness returned to the index finger at my tenth point. The intensity of the throbbing steadily diminished, and the pulses became less frequent. I concentrated on my breathing as, without really doing two things at once, I lowered my forehead pulse to match what was happening at his fingertip. He led me down and down until I was nearly dozing on my feet.

"Go find the silence," he suggested. I pictured him kneeling on his mat by the target, his eyes closed, his breath shallow. I now knew what he did at these times to prepare himself for the exertion of shooting. Most people flex and stretch their muscles to warm up; he slowed himself down.

We walked together for awhile and discussed the principle of doing the opposite of calisthenics. When we reached the stream he went out into the woods and I returned to the stone house and the target area. I unrolled his straw mat and knelt down—as I had often seen him do—with my knees on the ground and my legs pressed together beneath me. As I did this, I could imagine him inside me. This inner vision led me to act even more like him, with a great deal more knowledge about what he did internally than I'd had when I arrived. An image helps the student to approximate the master's composure, but to duplicate it one must do the internal adjustments that produce the external picture.

I rested my palms on my knees and slowly drew them up my thighs while letting my head float until it felt almost weightless. Then I forced myself to exhale as long as I could stand it. Taking a cue from my heart rate as it increased at the end of the exhale, I generated the ten pulses one at a time. Each point demanded attention and then a flexing of the adjacent channels to push it forward. When I completed the task, and the pulse in my forehead felt as if it were shooting sparks, I began shortening my exhales. My breath became more even and quiet, and my heartbeat quieted, the rate slowing as if I were falling asleep. This must be some sort of self-hypnosis, I thought.

Regulating the pulses is more than self-hypnosis, though; it is also a means of controlling the ki vibrations. The lower they become, the more the ki surrounds the body as if diffused throughout the immediate atmosphere. The stronger the pulses become, the more they concentrate the ki in the body's diamond. To find harmony with the environment before some exertion, one must slow the pulse rates in the wells of ki to gain the maximum skill.

The stillness I attained on the mat by the target was very different from ordinary silence. This stillness had many gradations, like musical scales. At the end I felt as though

I were drawing strength in from outside myself. Actually, I was in a transition mode from the normal efforts of moving about to the exertion of drawing the bow. Yet, in this meditative transition stage I established a space where the external world was silenced into the womblike cocoon of self-containment. The erratic pulse in the groin caused by kneeling soon became a steady ticking like a watch and, finally, a warm flow along the channels surged into the spine. I felt indestructible. Maybe this diffusion of the ki is what the masters mean by inner peace.

The process of raising all the pulses and then lowering them took about twenty minutes, an appropriate period of time for most meditations. I reported all my discoveries to the master, who told me that the more I did this, the better. I would, he claimed, reach a state where just entering the powershift would evoke the ki source of the pulses. He could have told me never to try shooting without such a transition, but I was already convinced that some version of sitting on the mat would have to become part of my own ritual if I were to succeed in shooting arrows from horseback or doing anything with the kind of graceful motions the master had.

1 0

FEAR OF FALLING

At night I wondered what it might be like to be the master. While the stationary archer usually has a different perspective from that of a walker, runner, or rider, the master maintained his inner stillness during even the most arduous movements, as if his life's training was intended to bestow on him mastery of motion. He claimed that I should be able to shoot just as well riding as standing still. He advised me against looking for anchors outside of the self. There is no need for sights and a fixed position with a Zen arrow. I had to practice blending my mind-body with the terrain when riding or shooting. To find this continuum, the rider sets the ten points of his diamond and lets his eyes feed his Diamond Being rather than his thoughts.

The forest area the master chose to train my intuitive ability in the powershift was steep, twisting, narrow, and filled with loose logs and protruding branches. It looked neither safe nor passable, so how could I avoid looking outward? As a result, the master got so far ahead of me that I couldn't ask him for help. By anticipating the hidden difficulties, I also failed to trust the horse, thus borrowing trouble.

The rain clouds had lingered overnight, leaving us with

a humid, drizzly morning and slippery ground. Since I couldn't see my teacher on the trail and I didn't know whether he was waiting for or watching me, I was eager to prove myself. I warned myself to use my reflexes to pull myself forward. (In the East, I imagined, they pull themselves forward, whereas we tend to push ourselves onward.)

Entering the Diamond Being, through the powershift motions I became a kind of geometric creature with psychic powers, able to force the intuition to overcome rational fears. The quick moves of the horse showed me why the master had trained me to take this tack. The problem is simple enough. There is not enough time to draw a bow, point an arrow, and release the shot without being prepared to do so. Somewhere ahead is a target as well as an instant from which it is possible to line up with that target. The arrow must be released at a precise moment, which the horse traverses in one single stride.

On the narrow trail I had to react quickly, without thinking about where the horse might falter, and yet move with a sense of the free space existing between the present danger and future pitfalls. I did so by keeping my breathing in the pattern that allowed the mind to slow down enough to be intuitively alert. I envisioned a path through the branches and amplified the slow motion by chanting simple syllables. This technique broke the trail into safe, manageable segments. It also created a ghost that existed seventeen seconds into the present. The horse and I slowly plunged ahead through the juniper, like animated cartoon characters. After ten minutes, we wove between two more branches, passed between three more boulders, and lo and behold reached the pasture. The master was sitting quietly on his horse chewing on a grass stalk.

As I approached him, he raised the reins, sprang forward with a yell, and began zigzagging down the slope. The horse was neither walking nor running; his white legs pranced while his torso glided effortlessly against the backdrop of trees. I let my horse move at a pace just over the edge of my sense of safety and gave up any concern about injury. I loped along, inspired by the master's practiced movements. My intuitive faculty was calculating at a speed faster than I could think. I exhaled against my tanden, crouched slightly, and was swept along. This sudden ease at such a downhill speed was unexpected. I was riding fast and seeing myself in slow motion.

We could stumble without falling, our pace and rhythm propelling us without any conscious intervention. Then, where the horse ran frequently and the long grass trapped water, I saw innumerable mudholes. This change in the ground caused me to turn cautious, and suddenly I slid back into a normal consciousness in which I had a choice between slowing down and speeding up. I bent forward in the saddle, the spell of my riding meditation broken. I had to dismount in the midst of the bog, then trudge out with my tail between my legs.

I could discourse at length on the difference between riding with inner stillness and riding haphazardly. While the inner stillness existed, so did the continuum with the terrain. Once I lost concentration on the Diamond Being my abnormal abilities ceased. I had come down the slope gracefully, but not in my ordinary state of mind: I was lost inside the Diamond Being. This absence of any other self is the secret of Zen motion.

I became acutely aware of the value of the master's approach: he made no distinctions based on the difference in tasks. It didn't matter that I had no bow in my hands; I was learning how to enter a complex presence by ignoring space and time. I recognized some of the qualities of the presence, but I was far from understanding it. Of all my work with the master, the sense of becoming a Diamond Being was the most fascinating. The master had other names for this experience that were more philosophical. I didn't have any other way of translating them, especially since emptiness was a hard concept to make as tangible as the Diamond Man.

Three days passed before I dared return to the field's edge to review what had happened. At the place where I'd broken through the foliage, I spent twenty minutes reaccustoming myself to the landscape. I recalled the route the master had used to zigzag his horse down the slope and made a mental hologram of the master riding, then set it in motion. I could feel him riding and envision his Diamond. No one actually sees the Diamond's ten-point lattice; rather, one feels, by intuition, the complex presence. This, he says, is the correct envisioning—as opposed to the didactic internal movie-making common to Westerners. He doesn't see himself; rather, he feels the action of gravity around him. The weakness of the movie image is its very normalcy; it robs us of our subconscious ability to discern reality in dimensions accurate enough to do something as complex as shooting a bow from a horse.

On my return to the field I was newly aware that

concentrating enough to feel a presence is much harder than visualizing an image. One distraction and, even if I were sitting on the ground, I reverted to seeing a photograph of the master riding. By using my intuitive memory, glancing ahead but scanning rather than viewing the slope, I suddenly saw what had happened the other day. I had turned and cut back on the slope every twenty seconds in accord with my normal breathing pattern. He had done so every forty seconds. The sly fox gauged distance by his breathing, knowing full well that I would come up twenty yards short of where he reached the pasture because my breath was too short to avoid the bog. He was letting me know that I was self-satisfied and not improving the length of my exhale. I was working on too many things at once.

As a result of my constant walking and riding in the powershift, I kept waking up with ki spasms in my ankles; they would start twitching under the covers. These tiny explosions lasted about as long as the pain of hitting the funny bone. My very flesh was reacting to the heel-to-heel style of walking and to keeping the heel below the stirrup when riding. I had been inclined to believe in mind over matter, but day by day I was changing my views, and I was *seeing* mind in matter. In this way I began to correctly envision what it would be like riding down the slope with my bow drawn, rising to point the arrow at the target, and releasing the string without any fear of falling. I was beginning to see this still amorphous shape that I would become when he finally let me mount with my bow in hand.

1 1

B A L A N C E

In the first part of my training, my practice had to do with observing what is subtly contained in the powershift. Under the master's guidance I had developed the skills needed to observe the mind-body connections in great detail. One day he determined that I was ready for the next stage. He said that the further refinement of the powershift depends on balance, and balance depends on centering oneself by intricate stance work on the spine and its curves. For him, centering wasn't a psychological activity. He taught balance and centering by an ultra-slow walking meditation that requires altering the central nervous system's awareness of ki.

He showed me again that, when unstrung, his long bow resembled a human spine. The bow, he claimed, is the only tool needed to balance the channels of the Diamond Being. His bow of laminated bamboo, called a *yumi*, had four designated curves: the princess curve, corresponding to the neck and shoulders; the bird curve, corresponding to the hump of the thorax; the inward curve, corresponding to the concave indent at the small of the back; and the little curve, representing the coccyx.

With the resemblance to the spine noted, he handed me the bow he'd been breaking in—a bow filled with his

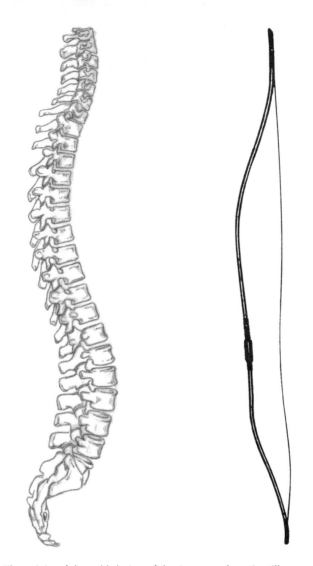

*The origin of the odd design of the Japanese bow is still a puzzle
for scholars. The almost exact relationship to the shape of
the spine has led the archers to a doctrine of inner and outer
equilibrium. For the Easterner, the way the coccyx acts
as a mirror image to the lower tip of the bow can represent
the yin and yang rather than a contradiction of form.*

BALANCE   **75**

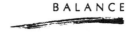

efforts. He took his other, suppler bow and bid me follow him. We took a winding path through the pine woods to a dirt road leading to a small pavilion with a plank floor. I followed his step as best I could. The pavilion was made of stone, glass, and unfinished wood. By contrast, the wood of the bamboo bow was polished to perfection. Its staff was very long compared to a Western bow but extremely lightweight. Its end was delicate, and I dared not let it touch the road.

Under the pavilion I was quite aware of being alone with him. "This is another, more serious form of walking meditation that I am about to show you," he says.

He drew himself into the breath posture, adjusting his shoulders and belly, placing his feet in the same stance as if he were going to shoot an arrow. This time, however, he held the bow at arm's length in front of him. Concentrating fiercely on this staff, he slowed his breathing down to two inhalations per minute. I watched, yet to do so with any understanding I had to imitate him.

With his example to inspire me, I regulated my breathing to three inhalations per minute. He closed his eyelids down to narrow slits and placed his feet close together, heel to toe. As I narrowed my vision I was aware of an intensifying contrast between light and shadow. In the breeze, the branches cast oscillating shadows. His head bobbed slightly, as though he were floating on his back in water. After three or four minutes, he moved his right foot around in front of his left. He slid his bow forward and paused again. I could barely restrain myself to match his glacialy slow pace.

When should I swing my right heel around to my left

toe? I assume it must be done as the breath begins to decline and the belly shrinks toward normalcy. This would be the steadiest instant. But I found standing with my feet in line rather awkward after a few minutes, and I started to lose balance. I wavered to the point where a slight blow from his bamboo shaft would have knocked me over. He didn't seem to notice how tentative I was. I kept changing the position of my shoulders and my head to steady myself. It took several tries to balance my upper torso so that I was steady when the breath was at the right stage. Without a conscious command to move, I just moved my foot because I was ready. It was akin to releasing the arrow when it was lined up with the target.

As my foot moved ahead, my arm stretched forward, using the bamboo as a counterweight. Light as it was, after holding the bow in front of me for four minutes, its weight became significant. I walked right behind the master as, ever so slowly, we traversed the thirty-foot circumference. The tension rose in my spine, and it grew harder and harder to keep my backside in the out-curved position the bow suggests.

I worked through the early pain, and by the second go-round I had relaxed. My Diamond Being was watching me from a distance, and it saw that I was becoming the bow. The realization was somewhat eerie, and thus the ki moved more rapidly along my spine. My locked hips kept the concave shape in my lower back, and my tucked chin kept the back of my head straight. By the third circling I felt the ki's power intensify within.

With each step I became better at waiting for balance to occur suddenly at the moment of stillness. The bamboo staff acted as a level—something like mercury seemed to be rising and falling inside it. I actually felt the arc of ki go above and below me, or, as the master says, "You feel the thread that holds the bow between heaven and earth." This thread curves slightly, like a drawn bow.

The master has said, "Breathing in unison, we cannot be distracted. A warming sensation fuses our spines. A cocoon envelops us; we walk as one with all the others."

I couldn't have made sense of these words without feeling the actual resonance of the ki between my bamboo staff and my spine. The arc that is abstract in concept is very real in practice. The cocoon that envelops is an aspect of the complex presence. Mine was especially tangible because it had become entwined with his. As I imitated him, his slightest move was transmitted psychically. The pace became easier to maintain, and I didn't need to move the next foot right away because there was pleasure in resting and waiting for him to trigger the move. An osmosis was taking place between us, the cocoon being formed by the very connection between us that synchronized our steps. This resembled what happened when we rode together: he triggered, I emulated, and the combined effort was greater than either's part. My intuitive sense of balance was being controlled by the sensations in my spine, which caused the ki to increase. This seemed peculiar to me, as it would for any Westerner imprisoned within linear, cause-and-effect beliefs: the ki should cause balance, not be co-extensive with it. What I had discovered was a mesh between the subjective and the objective world. The bow and the spine, the master and the pupil, all were joined by the similarity in their form and by the mysterious resonance.

The strange coincidence of ki and balance caused two images to float into my mind. I saw a black pool of oil with waves in concentric circles and then striated layers of rock in which the colored bands ran off into infinity. Every so often my Diamond Being caught a reflection of myself on the surface of the pool. I knew my sense of selflessness rippled in that blackness, and I wanted to immerse myself there. I perceived details—a nail bent in the post, a beetle, three stones in a line—as mere shapes in the void, without any sense of their setting. Oddly, self-containment left me more open than had my lackadaisical reality.

I grew lightheaded; my normal impatience decreased as my internal feel for the patterns of the field of life increased. A shimmering silence surrounded everything. I felt the shimmer because the master's Diamond Being had made me receptive to the universal flux; this supersensitive, antennalike state derived from having adjusted my spine to match the bow's shape. No doubt about it, inner balance—hence the level of ki—depended on the degree of vibration in the spine.

The mystic's secret is this heightened sensitivity. Spiritual healers actually feel the ki vibrations and the inner balance of their patients. Although they possess skills beyond my own, I could finally understand their receptiveness, the way their spinal system held the ki. Perhaps this sensitivity would be my natural state if I kept developing the Diamond Being.

I wasn't so narrowly focused on archery that I could not see that adjusting the spine had other ramifications. An improved powershift changes attitude by extending the range of possibility for both feeling and action. A master retains this level of sensitivity while riding a horse. A master can even know another person's level of awareness by observing posture and stance. It makes sense, because the brain and the spine are more connected within the Diamond Being, and therefore the full human potential is utilized, allowing paranormal abilities to become ordinary.

1 2

THE INTUITIVE FEEL

I have always prided myself on my ability to observe details, never admitting that there were observations I often missed because of my individual mind-set or because I am from a particular culture. For instance, it would never have occurred to the master to wonder why the arrow isn't shot on a straight line. I thought that you shoot on a high line and let the arrow drop over distance. "But no, never; the arc of ki is always curved," he exclaimed. "You must shoot so that the arrow drops through the target." The changing of a mind-set needn't be a slow process. Once the new knowledge is implanted one should commence using it. His statement gave me an idea, and I was ready to start using the feel of the curve in my practice.

I gave myself the assignment of jumping from one bank of the stream to the other. I chose an area where the width was slightly beyond my ability to jump. It was in a wooded spot a few hundred yards east of my cabin. Branches and brush shielded my efforts from others. I wasn't going to improve my physical prowess overnight, but I hoped to improve my ability to sense the arc of ki in the jump.

I squatted in the tall grass and assembled my ten points into the powershift, quieting my mind by concentrating on pushing the tanden out as far as possible on each long exhale. As soon as my heart pulsations increased I focused on the point on the opposite bank where I would have to land in order not to sink into mud. I gave myself plenty of time to gather my resources by setting my attention on each point of the diamond. I envisioned the jump completed by my being pulled forward and landing above the mud line. My muscles tensed with strength; I had to wait until the adrenalin subsided and the muscles in my legs relaxed. In a few minutes I slowed down the pulses in the ki wells. In this calm, I assessed how far I might be able to spring forward in a single leap. In the air above the water I located an imaginary dot at the height I needed to achieve to reach the other side. This is the same dot an archer would use in calculating the apex of an arrow's arc. It takes an extra effort to notice it, yet the distance of the jump or the arrow depends on finding it.

I figured out how to place my feet and my weight and how much to bend my knees to intuit the apex. I wanted a track coach to come guide me, but then it occurred to me that since childhood I had lost any sense of working with the Diamond Being, relying instead on physical ability. An on-your-mark-get-set-go attitude had blinded me to the single critical part of the action: the concentration on the split second before it begins. To leap at random was to miss the apex; to leap after having concentrated through the pain of holding the ready-to-jump crouch five or six seconds more than usual was to sail across and hence through the jump.

Increasing my ability required bringing the wells of ki to their full pulsations. I changed the way I observed myself.

Instead of thinking about how to jump, I was paying attention to the stillness inherent in the moment prior to the leap and feeling ki momentum build. (The Zen archer also does this when shooting an arrow from a horse. The jumper's crouch or squat is similar to the position in the saddle, and the same moment of stillness characterizes the approach to the target.) A hurried shot from a horse will always go awry. I should jump or shoot only when my mind couldn't concentrate the effort any longer. By the act of concentrating to the limit I was achieving patience. Telling myself to be patient and not to jump too soon only caused anxiety, but if I looked for the arc I had something specific to do that took time.

At the stream, I wasn't calculating the jump but waiting for the trajectory to become clear to me. The moment this happened I knew when to release. At the split second the arc appears, the jump takes place with a feeling of certainty. If I leapt in order to reach the other bank, I wasn't concentrating on the specific task of reaching the apex of the arc—which, incidentally, was easier than trying to leap the stream. When I fell from the height of my jump I caught a foothold on the opposite bank. To go across on sheer momentum required a running start and a jerky landing. I began to see why the master's arrows penetrated deeper than mine did: he shot with the arc.

"You must be governed from within," the master would say, and he reinforced this lesson each time we gathered to watch him shoot his bow. He had a tremendous ability to concentrate the ki abiding in the ten wells of his Diamond Being into the shot. The strongest arrows seemed to be propelled by more than just the bow. The air became charged when he shot, filled with the vibrations of the taut string and body.

A Western observer would be caught up in watching what he was doing and how he was doing it, and thereby miss the thing he was demonstrating—the when of the shot. Students are often caught up in the complicated how-to of Zen archery, but he seemed concerned only with timing, with the moment when the arc of ki is in the open window. The arrow must be shot then, and shot through the bull's-eye rather than at it. Otherwise, the arc is not completed and the arrow fails to penetrate deeply.

When some of the less experienced students shot, I would feel that their timing was off, that they released too abruptly, before the real window of opportunity opened. The training of my intuition was more advanced than theirs, and I could feel that the complex presence they needed to attain wasn't complete. As I felt their incompleteness, so the teacher felt mine, and his master felt his. The target is completeness, not the bull's-eye, and thus where the arrow lands is irrelevant. A perfect shot can occur even if the string breaks and the arrow falls to the ground—if the archer reaches the point of completeness and the window of the arc opens. To the trained ear, the window opens with a sharp crack.

I must make it clear that my teacher starts pulling his bow with his arms over his head, so that it grows taut as the arms reach shoulder level. The bow bends far above his head since the arrow is shot from below the midpoint of the bow. Once having attained this dynamic, he stands under such great tension that his bow hand wavers and his abdomen bulges and ripples. Even so, his breath remains calm and steady as his mind seeks the arc. There is a pause, a kind of long second, and then he concentrates his attention on his hand as it draws the string back an inch more. His bow wavers in a jerky motion that appears awkward to Western eyes. As he waits for the feel of the the arrow's arc to the target to center in his tanden, he completes the exhale, and the arrow disappears in a great shout. The shout is the echo of the window opening.

At full draw no one can hold the hand steady using a six-foot bamboo bow and a thirty-six-inch arrow. Even the master cannot aim precisely. But he is able to feel the moment when the instant is right for the release, and he lets go without any hesitation. On horseback he must actually suspend time for an instant just before he pushes his right hand back. This still instant is necessary to allow him to perceive the arc. Each perception is one of many rapid connections or jumps that are the hallmark of those on the path of intuition. There are many little revelations, not one major revelation. Each one is a surprise and each is a gift. The master bows to the target and withdraws.

The Western archer shooting at or from moving targets has to decide when to release the arrow to compensate for the motion. The archer can attempt to rely on reflexes or on lining up the sight pin and the bull's-eye, but it is very difficult to do this quickly enough to be sure of oneself. The Zen master relies on the intuition of his Diamond Being. A Westerner thinks this being is an abstraction, while the trained student thinks it is the only concrete reality one can trust. Hence, there are believers and doubters.

The believers feel that muscular, reflexive aiming doesn't

train the mind-body to reach the zenith of the intuitive feel. They say that only with the unfettered mind and the discipline of concentration in the adjusted stance can it be transferred from one activity to another. These believers say that, since a master depends on the intuitive feel, he can shoot in the dark or on uneven terrain where sights are useless, that he can shoot an invisible arrow with an envisioned bow. The doubters say that the only proof is in the location of the real arrow in the target.

I can reply to the doubters only with the following account.

Every time the master releases an arrow his right arm flies back from the bow and stops with his elbow straight back and his forearm at a ninety-degree angle to it, and his hand vibrates for five seconds. It shakes from the wrist like a quivering leaf. To watch this manifestation of the ki in a person is the only absolute proof of its existence.

One day I said to him, "This long vibration of the hand doesn't happen when anyone else shoots."

The teacher scratched his neck and looked up at me, his left eye squinting as he tilted his head. "After I shoot, it isn't my hand anymore," he said. "Sometime, I will show you why."

I waited three days for him to invite me to the target range. So many aspects of daily living intervened that I became impatient. New visitors came, and they further distracted him from archery. It wasn't until I was engrossed in my own practice one day that he unexpectedly appeared along the stream.

I pulled an arrow back as far as I could, and it swerved down into the ground and bounced up under the target.

He didn't seem surprised. I was too aware of the physical bow, he claimed.

"After you go back as far as you can with your arm's strength, you must concentrate your mind on the further draw of the arrow. It will seem impossible to pull more. But as you concentrate and breathe, ki will *push* the hand back on the taut string with a slow stretch. Eventually, you will forget your muscles and the Diamond Being will hold the bow for you."

That evening he wrote this verse and gave it to me.

> The Rainbow behind the bow.
> The Silence behind the string.
> The Mind behind the arrow.
> This is the Way of the shaking hand.

The following series of illustrations shows the archer's practice with the underlying powershift.

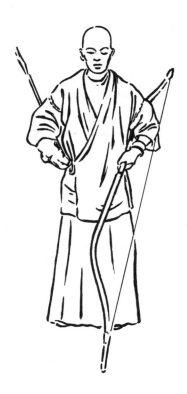

The archer prepares himself for shooting by first relaxing in a normal stance, looking down at the ground and inviting the weight of his mental tension to fall toward the ankles.

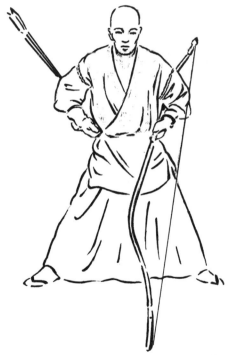

*Spreading the feet wide braces the body. The archer looks at the
ground to focus his attention inward.*

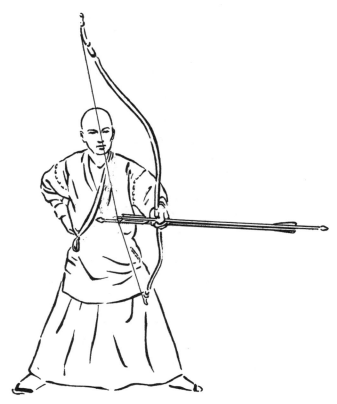

*The coccyx is drawn back, causing the shoulders to come forward.
The abdomen is relaxed. Notice that there are two arrows on the
bow, one facing away and the other facing toward the archer.
These preparatory actions are ritualized; they do not
resemble anything done in western archery.*

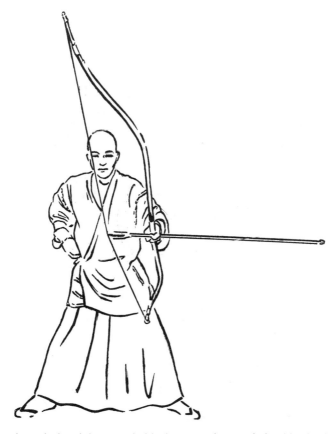

The right hand that now holds the second arrow behind his back reminds the archer to excursion his hips and lock the lower back in an indented position. While the archer's posture looks the same as in the last drawing, his skeletal alignment is completely different.

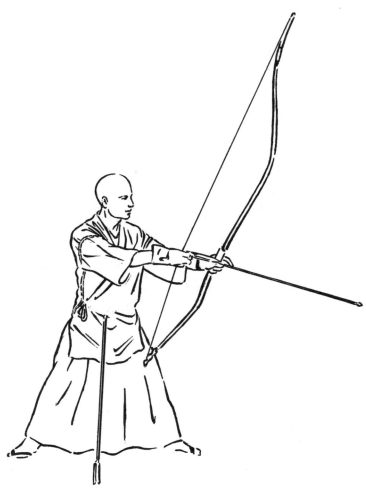

*When attention is turned to the target, the archer bends back
from the sides, allowing his belly to protrude. The second
arrow is placed at his belly and extends to the ground.*

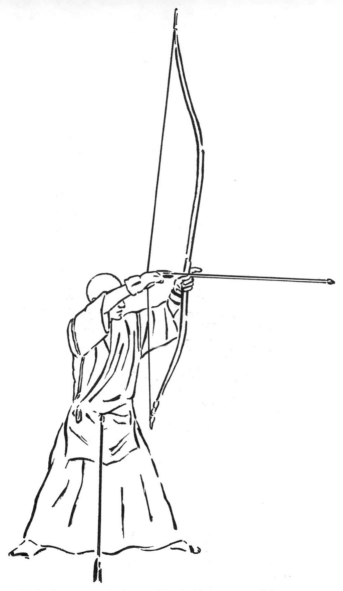

The belly is expanded enough to hold the point of the arrow despite the upward movement of the arms because the breath is being directed downward to the tanden. The shoulders are raised without rotating them back as the archer moves the bow above his head.

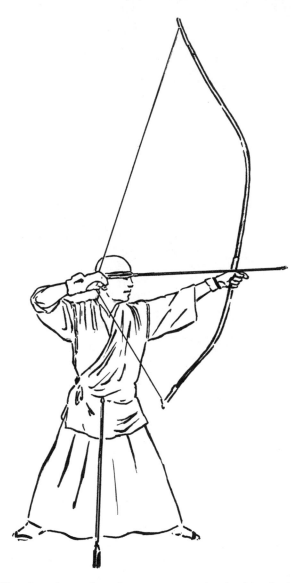

Pulling the string to draw the arrow rotates the shoulders back, causing the upper spine to curve backward. Drawing the bow from above the head inclines the body forward.

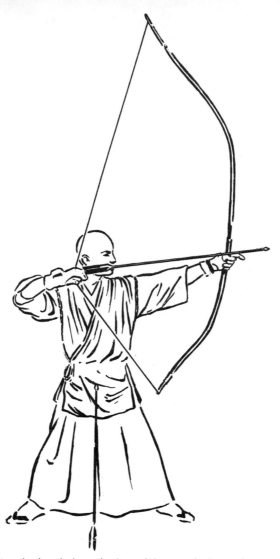

Pulling the hand along the line of the mouth draws the arrow all the way back, creating the same change in posture as pressing the shoulders down in the powershift. The ki energy in the shoulder wells is martialed for this final bend of the bow. The shoulders must press down to hold the arrow from drifting forward. At full draw the belly is totally extended to help hold the tension of the bow at the center of the body.

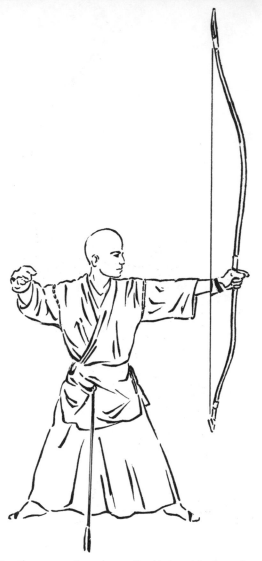

Releasing the arrow also releases the ki stored in the spine. This allows the archer to keep the hand from shooting backward; instead, the hand vibrates a few inches behind the point of release. The tension of bow and body are released but also absorbed and controlled. The direction of the arrow is determined by the timing of the release and the line of breath that is expelled.

1 3

STILLNESS IN MOTION

My teacher insisted that I shouldn't shoot my bow from a horse before practicing the concentration on driving the string hand away from the target. His admonitions made no sense to me. I knew that falling off a horse while holding a bow and arrow could cause injuries, but I had planned to go at the task cautiously. I didn't suspect that the motion that drives the arrow hand back also balances the rider on the horse while shooting. An equal and opposite reaction to the force of the shot does not unbalance the rider.

Moving the hand back by concentrating the mind on it is difficult, but the powershift holds a reserve of the ki's resonant energy. Stretching the ki channels releases this reserve—and it makes no difference whether the student thinks of this as normal muscle energy or ki power. The effect is that the hand overcomes the pull of the string and begins to fly back upon release. When the student becomes a master, his hand will vibrate with the abundance of ki.

The master was eventually satisfied that I wouldn't hurt myself by just trying to ride with a bow. I prepared the area by raking the loose turf and picking up rocks. I oriented myself to the target, which had been set on a gentle slope about fifteen feet above the cleared area. The actual arrangement was a T shape. We would ride along the top of the T and release the arrow from the side of the horse at the point of intersection. The target itself was simply a rug draped over the top pole of a children's swing set. Tacked on the rug were three small foam discs. The distance was forty yards.

I patiently watched the master's arrows against the grey sky of an overcast day in late summer. He brought the bow from over his head down to his shoulders, and the arrows dropped into the discs. Above us, the mountains were holding the outer edge of a hurricane from the Sea of Cortez, but there was no more rain left in the clouds.

When he finished, he brought the Indian Paint to the intersection point and tethered him. He lengthened the stirrups for me while I shot a few arrows to warm up. An archer can ride virtually bareback except for stirrups. It's the stirrups that provide the footing for long-range shooting. Stirrups were not introduced to the West until the Mongols rode into Europe in the Middle Ages.

The master listened to the sound my arrows made hitting the rug. After I had shot three strong ones in a row, he motioned for me to mount. My first task was to shoot the bow from a standstill, which I assumed would be pretty easy. With legs braced in the stirrups I could adjust my stance to draw the bow from above my head and then, bringing it down by stretching with both arms, I kept the bow from hitting either the horse's neck or the saddle. The effort of keeping my shoulders pressed down and my back curved held me straight in the saddle. Pushing breath against my tanden forced the center of gravity low enough to relax my upper torso. And, just as the master had said, concentrating on driving the right hand away from the target prevented any unbalanced leaning.

After my first shot, the training I had received suddenly took on a whole new significance: what had been slow, tedious, and strained on the ground became elegant on the horse. I had been given my wings.

Years of practice with a bow can produce great skill in a marksman, and although this skill can be glorified by the camera, it pales in comparison to the feeling of inner stillness that comes when the shot follows a practiced form. The body-mind acts in a patterned gracefulness with nary a thought. The powershift not only anchored me to the horse, it aimed and controlled the shot. The surprise turned out to be that I was good at shooting from a mounted position without ever having done it before.

In the alternative means of training, the sink-or-swim approach of Western society, I would have had to learn to pull the bow from horseback by trial and error. The master would have had to coach me on what to do to aim an arrow. I suppose I would have improved bit by bit as the days went on, but by forcing me to remain on the ground to practice my breath-posture and stance-attitude, the master gave me this gift of fitting into the preexisting pattern of the Diamond Being and finding complete repose.

My elation subsided as the master led the horse in a fast walk perpendicular to the target. I faced the new problem of shooting while moving, one that is nearly impossible to anticipate. The only preparation is learning how to slow down the breathing to counter the stress of motion.

I rushed the first shot, but as I discovered the wisdom of

aiming by driving the shooting hand back along the arc of ki, my timing returned. Although each sway of the horse changed the angle of the shot, I adjusted my hand on the string immediately without moving the bow. I could detect the change in the trajectory and rapidly move my hand to trace it.

Intuition is the rapid, subconscious cross-checking that occurs when the ordinary mind doesn't intervene. The Diamond Being knows that the line to the target laid out by the laws of trigonometry also has a metaphysical shepherd in the arc of ki. An accurate shot occurs when the eyesight is subordinated to the workings of the intuition. The arc is felt in a flash; the archer at full draw waits for this inner flash. He realizes that if he lets go before it happens, the arrow will be off line. He adjusts his right hand in accord with his eyesight, forces it back against the target, and when the tension seems unbearable the arc appears. It's apex is discovered within the confines of the Diamond Being, which compensates for the up-and-down motion of the horse. The channels adjust to it, and with the breath nearly exhausted, the split second of the release draws out into an eternity. The archer's breath explodes from the tanden and, as the hand flies back, the breath flies forward to the target. After release, the inner spring uncoils through the body as the tension uncoils in the bow's limbs.

What I am describing is the sensation of an arc of action, not a line drawn in the sky like a jet's trail. The sensation is as concrete as the throbbing of a wound. We experience it at airports when a plane taxis up the runway and the adjacent plane seems to be moving, or when a car moves in the opposite direction to a train standing next to it. We automatically correct for the distortion in the motion.

I am stating the problem in the negative here, for just as you feel the unease of the distortion, you can feel the ease of alignment. The same physical vertigo takes place, but now it is compensated for by the Diamond Being. You can let a feeling of height cause you to fall or you can let it keep you balanced on a ledge. If you slow down anxiety, breathe in rhythm, and center in the ten-point stance, you will feel the balance necessary to move without falling. This balance is the arc of ki. It's the cat's leap, the arrow's flight, the problem's solution. Hit the right spot on the floor and with eyes closed you can drop the ball into the basket.

When the arrow's actual trajectory and the inherent arc of the shot discovered by the form coalesce (a sensation hard to put into words because of the resulting explosion) the world changes instantly, for in this explosion the whole isn't broken into parts—the parts become a whole. The stillness at the heart of motion—the Zen in motion—is revealed. Horse and rider move against the horizon and yet are stationary against an even larger backdrop.

One famous master pointed to the cranes in the sky and asked his student, "Where are they flying?"

"They have already flown away," came the reply, and the master twisted the student's nose. For a moment the student saw nothing, then he discovered the stillness in motion: the cranes in the sky were frozen in a painting, going neither south nor north. The master said, "They have always been here."

In the introduction I promised to refrain from preaching any kind of system; there are many paths, and each person finds his own. What counted most in my training wasn't the bow or the horse but the approach to learning. I am sure that there are athletes who, given sufficient incentive, could easily outshoot me with a bow from a horse or from the ground, and I would like to watch such a performance out of curiosity or for entertainment. However, it is unlikely that I would plant myself at the athlete's doorstep and ask him to teach me to improve myself. I would have to be convinced that he had attained a higher degree of human awareness: he would have to know when to twist my nose so that I would discover the Sea of Origin, which is both flux and stillness. The point of release cannot be taught, only discovered.

To move in stillness and to be still in motion is the quintessential lesson to be learned. To practice with the horse and the bow is an attempt to live the lesson. One doesn't get better with practice, although, as one might expect, competency improves. Having a bad day may ruin the shot. One gets better by living the lesson and eliminating bad days. I find that I shoot my bow better when writing poems rather than prose; my mind is less restricted, more in touch with the field of life.

My practice sessions begin within the ordinary, prosaic frame of mind. Most of the arrows miss the target, and the hits are accidental, yet each miss serves to focus the attention. By the fifth round, most of the arrows are in the target, the ones in the bull's-eye representing moments of harmony with the cosmic flux. The hour of archery practice is also an hour of meditation that transforms the archer by releasing the tensions that hold back the natural indwelling force.

As I shot the last arrows from the horse, I had conquered

nothing, won at nothing, mastered nothing, yet I was invincible for I was not *I* but *it*, the stillness in motion before the explosion. In a way, the beauty of the master's lesson is that it is imbedded in the practice. Stop practicing and you lose the ability to follow the arc of ki into the window of opportunity. The spontaneity of the last shot must be carried into the next activity, and the archer mustn't gloat over the strong shots or mourn the weak ones. Some connections and jumps may be wrong, but all the efforts toward interpenetration with the Sea of Origin are to be treasured.

1 4

SPEED AND TIMING

The day after my first shots from the horse, the master watched from the hillside as I practiced. Since I wasn't accustomed to riding without reins, I first rode the little Paint around the track using knee pressure to guide her before I remounted with a bow. With the reins draped over the horse's neck, I eventually managed to arrange the arrow and the bow. To increase the pace meant fitting into the horse's strides. I wasn't fully prepared for this, yet my willing attitude and novice's attention led to what is called "beginner's mind."

In effect, the master was no longer the teacher; I'd been turned over to his horse, Aj-o, who knew what was expected. It might even be said that this horse was the master's alter ego. Aj-o quickly noted that I was much less agile than his master. He would look back at me and shake his head in dismay whenever my shifting weight thwarted his movements. He'd been trained to move along until he heard the arrow release. He would wait to hear the next arrow nock on the string before resuming. I could trust him to be consistent, as long as I kept my mind on what I was doing, repeating the process in just the same way each time. In my youth any such discipline had made me rebel; now I considered it rewarding. We do change over time.

From a practical standpoint, the crux of shooting at a target positioned to the side of the horse is to release the arrow the second after passing the line to the bull's-eye, so that one is always shooting back against the motion of the horse. Around fifty pounds of pull is necessary to keep the arrow from drifting. The poundage of the pull is determined by the thickness of the bow's limbs and the distance the arrow is drawn back. Commonly, pull is measured at twenty-eight inches. A long bow allows one to pull back thirty-two or three inches; a short bow with stiffer limbs can reach fifty pounds at twenty-six inches. I soon discovered how hard it was to have the arrow drawn far enough back at the very second the horse pranced by the target.

Another way of stating the problem is to say that the archer must intuit both the trajectory and the speed before the horse runs past the target. Describing the objective this way leads the student into the interior work of breathing, setting the diamond posture, and envisioning the apex. Instead of trying to speed up the body, he slows down the perception. Correct timing occurs when he meshes the length of the exhale with the stride of the horse to arrive at the moment when the window for the shot opens. Ten rounds went by before I had a chance to release the arrow.

In the beginning, the horse was confused, but after a while I'd press his flanks and he'd speed up for the next shot. Aj-o would stop and I'd pull an arrow from the quiver, draw my shoulders back, squirm my coccyx back, and lock my body to the saddle in one motion. The arrow and bow were in my left hand as I raised myself upward. With my arms over my head, I drew the bow, simultaneously using a steady push pressure with my left arm and pull pressure with my right.

Each day the pull became easier. Aj-o, or my own horse, Chato, would stride parallel to the target and I would envision myself at the intersection, frozen in a moment of repose. As I came to full draw I sat back straight in the saddle, with the center of gravity in my belly. At the same time, I began pointing the arrow. My abdomen expanded, but the pressure at the tanden was much less than I could generate on the ground. I had to drive the tension down into the tanden so that my arm and shoulder muscles relaxed. Once they did, I could extend my neck and turn my face toward the target. The sense of the Diamond Being, that feeling of emptiness and concentration coupled to the flow of ki was critical, because it transferred my attention from external circumstances to the invisible plane on which the window opens.

There is no way to sight down the arrow shaft on a moving horse. The opportunity for a launch lasts about one-half of a second. There is no time to focus my eyes on the bull's-eye. The instant I see it before me is the instant I must release the arrow by thrusting the string hand away from my body. A thought delays the arrow too long; even opening the fingers causes a jerk on the string. And yet I must not hurry.

Being near the end of my exhale, my rib cage is flexible, and I lean to the left, extending the bow hand. The long arrow hangs five inches past the handle. I press my feet into the stirrups and, as I do, I can feel the horse go up and down under me. The target blurs, and I have to aim with the string hand by pulling the tension from my tanden.

The master says this action forms a cross of peacefulness: the spine drives into the saddle, fixing a vertical line, while a horizontal line extends from the right elbow through the third eye to the left elbow and out to the target. This is the ideal form; when I duplicate it the arrow is held over my head. If I do it right, it's more like lobbing the arrow into the arc than driving it along a line. I think I am going to miss the target and the arrow hits because my normal perception is wrong, while my intuitive perception of the arc is true.

If I practiced by myself for a hundred years, I would never have stumbled on this method of shooting an arrow from a horse. I would have concentrated on the eye-hand coordination between the bow hand and the target. I wouldn't have worked on the right kind of knowing that sustains the inner self and the need for spiritual purpose.

The rendezvous with any target through the arc is a kind of knowing that tells you if you are following the right path in your life. The psychic-perceptual skill informs you that what you are doing lies along your karmic path. Extend the arc as far back or as far forward as you like, if you are off line the intuitive feeling will be dissatisfaction. Intuitive voices mustn't be ignored in favor of the practicality of ordinary mind; they come from a deeper place, beyond comprehension.

1 5

THE SHOUT

A visitor to the retreat who came for meditation lessons told me that the master's younger brother had married a Tibetan woman and was living in Tibet's high western plains, working as a ranch hand. I was surprised to hear that a man from Kyoto would leave the city to become a "cowboy." The master's own Asian saddle was evidence that he had connections to those who rode on the steppes.

Every year at a spring festival in Mongolia, the horsemen come together and hold archery contests. They use short bows and slant them to shoot over the horse's head while charging past a target. The arrows can split a piece of wood. The wooden bows with sinew-tied recurved limbs are accurate at forty or more yards. The Mongol tribesmen ride short-legged, shaggy ponies that move as though they are marching, and so there is less up and down motion to disturb the rider. While their technique is somewhat different, it is based on the same principles as that of Japanese archers, whose roots can be traced back to the steppes.

Such horsemen reached the outskirts of Vienna in the mid-thirteenth century, and for the first time Europeans heard the chorus of their shouts. Far from being the unorganized horde that movies depict, they were units of men in strict formation, wave upon wave. I cannot imagine pulling a bow weighing seventy pounds, but the shout . . . the shout I know intimately. It is not an Indian war whoop but a "kiai," a release of breath from a body in what might be called a shamanistic trance. Perfecting the shout is in effect perfecting the art of self-containment, and it is a challenge to both student and teacher. The shout of a master propels the arrow hard enough to penetrate a thick leather shield. There are varying degrees of ki resonance in the shout, and the legend is that the great masters could stun an opponent with the shout alone. Mastering the shout requires not only shooting the bow and breathing, but also turning the violent nature, the urge to kill, into something spiritual. This is an inner force that lingers and vibrates through the mountains like the sound of a great Tibetan prayer horn. The shout without this resonance of the ki is a fake, a forgery easy to detect.

One afternoon the master suggested I try using the Mongolian style of turning the bow on a slant and shooting over the horse's head.

"You were very good at squatting," the master suggested. "You will shoot better on the horse when you are squatting and facing forward."

He was reminding me of a part of the training that had come easily to me—so easily, in fact, that I had learned without ever realizing I was being taught. When I shot my short recurve bow at the master's straw target by the stream, he would squat, sitting on his heels, some seven yards in front of me. I thought he was just being courteous and not standing in my peripheral view. Hence, whenever he shot I would sit back on my heels with my hands resting on my knees. If I breathed evenly, this position became quite invigorating. My calf muscles ached for a few minutes, but afterward I had a pleasant spring in my legs. I got into the habit of squatting for a few minutes when I wanted to pull myself together and focus my ki. I paid attention to bringing the ten-point stance into perfect form by rotating my shoulders back and letting my head waver until it settled on my spine and helped me balance on my toes.

The master suggested I try practicing my shout from this position. "I don't think I can get much breath from this position," I said.

"Try," he encouraged.

I pressed my breath against the tanden, exhaled to the end, and made a noise like a puppy. The master came over and patted my head. "Start down in your heels. You are yelping from the chest. A good shout reflects a clear mind."

I had the image of pulling the shout up from the ground, amplifying it in the spring of my legs, and then expanding my abdominal muscles to force it out. At first, I made a weak noise, but at least it had some bass resonance. I practiced the shout for several days until I nearly lost my voice. This was evidence that I was doing something wrong.

"Use your hands as you try to shout," the master advised me, making a graceful gesture resembling a tai-chi movement. I asked him to do it a few more times.

He stretched his left arm in front of his face, then relaxed the wrist so that his fingers pointed at his eyes. He rubbed his thumb from the pinky to the index finger, generating more dexterity in the fingers. He then made a fist with his right hand and pointed it down toward his left hand from the height of his right ear. Wrists and elbows were both very loose.

He inhaled, pushing air into his mouth with his left hand. It was a brief gesture, and his eyes were intently focused on a nearby branch. I could tell that he was aiming his shout. His whole body concentrated, and the Diamond Being seemed almost visible for an instant, as his withdrawing left hand pulled the breath from his belly as though it were attached to a string. His right hand opened and arched backward in a beautifully relaxed motion. The two hands moved apart at the same speed, and his lips pursed, causing a square-jawed grin I'd seen just before he released an arrow. Just prior to full extension of his left arm, his right hand flew back, releasing the sharp crack of his kiai. I swear to this day that the branch moved as though in a sudden gust of wind. The sound reminded me of someone straining to lift a great weight, yet it traveled rapidly.

I waited a minute, then tried to duplicate his hand gestures. He was watching me and I was trying to get the gist of it. I got my hands into the position and wiggled my wrists. I started to exhale and move my hands apart. He shook his head sharply. Again, he demonstrated the motion for me. His hands didn't pull apart, they swooped away from each other in two curves. I nodded.

It was a lovely feeling, lifting my hands like bird's wings, slowly bringing the ki up into my lungs from the heels, and blowing air at my left hand. My fingers were linked by a long cat's cradle of invisible filament. I was pulling something apart, a sphere. There was a palpable ball, an expanding balloon. I could feel the breath dwindle in my

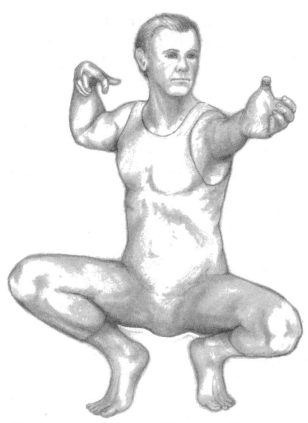

The shout resonates at nearly full extension of the arms, as the left shoulder is far forward and the right is thrust back. This twist faces the final burst of air, the kiai shout. The same twist underlies the Mongolian style of archery on horseback, the release of the arrow releasing the shout.

lungs and the balloon reach the point of bursting. The master smiled with some excitement. The shout would be the bursting of the balloon, a big pop that I could feel coming. Before I knew it the shout was over with. I heard my shout at a distance, as though it had no relation to me at all.

"At last," he said, "I don't have to grind teeth."

What he meant became clear as I tried the Mongolian style of shooting: it required the exact hand motions he'd shown me while I was squatting. I was opening the bow by uncurling my left arm in front of my face and pulling back with a fist above my right ear. Once the bow was in my hands these motions seemed obvious.

I faced the target ahead of me, with my weight distributed as if I were squatting rather than sitting. Chato and I were going slightly uphill, yet I didn't fall back as I pulled on the string because the uncurling left hand provided balance. I could feel the whole shot perfectly, being concerned with neither its inner nor outer form. The moment was all-encompassing. The arrow pulled back without any muscular effort; my wrists were as loose as could be. What had happened to the strain? I didn't have to aim or point, because the arrow would go wherever I blew my breath. The same gliding I'd achieved in my walk was now happening on horseback. The Mongolian style and the horse's motion felt perfectly harmonious.

I shouted in joy—spontaneously—and experienced a kiai without any strain. The window opened, revealing the arc of ki, a sixth-sense rainbow that began in the Diamond Being and extended through the target. The arrow released when I could pull back no more. Chato veered from the track and bounced on his hind legs. I never saw where the arrow hit until we retrieved it.

"This is your way," the master said. "Don't think you

can give up other training just because this is so."

I wasn't listening exactly. He was cautioning me that all the practice was what had made me capable, but he was also delighted that I'd done the whole procedure on my own. The real lesson was not in archery, though; it was a lesson in the method, for I had easily transferred from one style of shooting to another. Although the master had been training me to shoot with the bow held vertically, my predilection was for the slanted style. Finally there was something I could do with a touch of mastery. Had it been worth so much time and effort?

I was beginning to compare shooting arrows with writing books. There were books I wanted to write and books I was meant to write. What I wanted to do didn't turn out nearly as well as what seemed less practical but more fated. Of course, there was more effort expended than planned, since writing, like archery, had become for me a practice on the path of intuition. I knew what pages belonged to me alone; I had made peace with my strengths and limitations. Nearly fifty years old, I understood why the path of intuition could be termed the way of self-containment. I sympathized with my teacher's penchant for solitude and for finding true friendship through contact with fellow travelers. The best writing is done to teach oneself, to record the world in an intuitive grasp.

1 6

INTUITIVE HEALING

The repeated pulling of the bow from sometimes awkward angles while in motion, as well as the attempt to thrust the string hand away from the bow, makes archery a more dangerous activity for the body than one might expect. Even adepts forget themselves at times.

My injury resulted from an onslaught of zeal. I intended to improve my shooting ability to demonstrate for other students and wound up straining ligaments in my left arm so badly that I could hardly lift the bow four days later. A visitor heard my tale of distress and kindly offered her services. She was a thin, olive-complexioned woman with a British accent, the kind of person I believed would possess esoteric knowledge.

There were no formalities; I lay down on my bed and she knelt at my side. She passed her right hand over my left arm some eight inches above the flesh. She passed over a second time, then a third, moving her palm slowly along the afflicted area. At the end of her fourth pass she flicked her fingers as if trying to shake off a spider web. I felt nothing unusual and closed my eyes, expecting that this would take some time. Every now and then during a span of five minutes I opened my eyes and saw her moving her palm over my left elbow toward my thumb. I lay there in an idle doze, when suddenly I felt a searing flash of heat through the injured tendon. The rest of my arm felt normal. I made some kind of exclamation and sat up, raising my arm to examine it. The first thing I thought of was the older monk's statement about how body cells line up with the universal flux.

The heat had cured the tendon.

The woman told me she had used a therapeutic touch that she'd learned in New York. I thanked her profusely, since it was wonderful to be spared the pain. However, even though there was no pain under normal conditions, the problem was that I still couldn't use my bow; any attempt to pull it stretched the sore tendon. If I stopped, the pain stopped. I was fixed but not healed. My friend explained that when an injury occurs, the damaged cells become misaligned and therefore cannot resonate at the normal frequency. A person who can direct the ki into her hands has the capability of realigning cells. Theoretically, her cells acted like a tuning fork on my cells, and the searing heat that I felt had been caused by their sudden ability to resonate the ki again.

"If the ki is lacking, the area will be colder than normal," the master explained. "Your problem is that the cells' alignment is fine, but the tissue itself is still weak."

"Can I do anything to help heal the damage?"

"You are going to have to stop shooting for a while," he said, and I felt as though a sentence of banishment had been passed. "Of course, if this were a battle you couldn't rest very long. There is a means of increasing the ki in the injured area that builds up strength in the tissue."

After drinking three cups of green tea, he was prepared to demonstrate the means. I finished my second cup and sat with my back turned to him. We were underneath the canvas that shaded his favorite meditation area in the woods above the house—a small campsite with a log lean-to.

To speed the healing of my arm he first had to focus on my shoulder. It was a curious geometry and I was soon intrigued by the process. The same pulse that I'd felt in his finger when he touched my forehead was now being focused on the well of ki in my left shoulder. The well's pressure point is closer to the spine in the back and closer to the clavicle in the front. He told me that a ki well has a strong center pulse and four weaker satellite pulses. He probed around in my shoulder until he found the smaller points that responded to his finger pulse with pulses of their own. I could feel him exhale and press, causing a subtle feeling in which the effect came from duration rather than intensity. But soon my shoulder began pounding like a heart when one is running uphill; the other nine points seemed to feed this area. The master remained deep within himself, doing almost nothing that showed on the outside.

I could feel it when he stopped drawing on the ki in the atmosphere, but I had no idea how he determined when enough was enough. The stoppage was the result of a subjective determination, and a presence that had subtly insinuated itself ceased. By no means was there any transference of something inside him to me; rather, what was in and around me was focused through the ki channels while I was in a state of meditative stillness. The pulsations of gravity affect cells differently when we are still.

So many crazy theories about how intuitive healing works have been propounded that I am left with physical sensations I have few explanations for. My hunch is that the ki and gravity waves are related by the kind of contact with the Sea of Origin that many call interpenetration— and I'm just thankful for the healing power it offers.

Once he stopped focusing his efforts on me and entered into his own Diamond, I realized how much the esoteric secrets have to do with span of attention and subtle observation of detail. I had to focus on the Diamond's points and regulate pulses of ki, since my responsibility was to amplify his efforts. I couldn't work on myself until I engaged the powershift and quieted my breathing. I balanced my head, then drifted into the attitude of not-doing. He put his palm over the top of my head while, with his finger, he pressed the center pressure point in my shoulder.

He kept this up until the pulses in both areas had equalized at a level about half of what the shoulder pulse had been. As he worked, he rocked me slowly back and forth. I anticipated a jolt of searing heat, but instead I experienced an overall transformation that had no specific sensory component. It was more like a relaxation and cessation of weight.

The more I relaxed, the more the injured arm relaxed and thickened. I figured that more blood was flowing from my left shoulder down through my arm. I lengthened the time of exhale by three seconds and hummed to myself. My humming became a replication of a cat's purr and descended into my spine allowing some interesting adjustments. All together, these minute actions increased the strength in my arm. The lesson for healing damaged cells apparently mimed the lesson for shooting the bow: adjust the spine while exhaling in a slow, even breath and entering the Diamond Being.

I managed—or we managed—to generate the familiar twinges of the jarred funny bone, but this time they traveled the ridge through my tendon toward the the sensitive point in my palm, which the master was pressing gently with his thumb. The tissue was receiving more blood and oxygen, giving the cells the chance they needed to absorb the ki and rebuild the damaged areas. I really didn't know what the internal process was, but I ascertained that I had been hit by a powerful kiai. There was no sound, and yet an effect was caused as if there were sound. It was a kiai which, as when I was shooting the very best of arrows, went inward rather than outward, to the interior bull's-eye rather than the target. (Sometimes they are the same.) We Westerners tend to expect power to reside in volume. That the quality of the ki in the kiai could be volumeless and that a shout can be silent indicates how paradoxical the true physics of the ki is.

If I was prone to think this a miraculous technique that I could turn around and use on anyone, the state of the silence revealed the sobering truth: I couldn't tell if it was the master's kiai or my own. I'd had so much practice with the powershift that I was receptive to ki exchanges. Results are determined by composure and attention to the channels, not by willed intentions. Things like images, crystals, and icons are merely guides for the attention; more important is the preparation of the powershift.

I had been taught the Diamond Being's geometry from a master who had a perfect feel for the resonance of ki in others. His mastery is in his ability to detect the spirit of the mind-body, what the Japanese call *shin*. Accordingly, he is frequently asked to aid other masters in the dying process and so travels long distances to be with them. Awareness of the *shin* is what reconciles life and death into a similar phenomenon, because the *shin* is the indestructible part of the Diamond Being: it is the very thrust and expansion of the universe. Mystical experiences of this thrust cause the solid dichotomies of Western mental categories to vanish. It isn't that death and life are the same but that the continuum of the Diamond Being is on an unbroken string. It weakens during illness and dying, and thus we need help at these times to cast the line into the Sea of Origin.

I managed to continue the healing process by stopping for ten minutes every two hours—taking my medicine at regular intervals, so to speak. Instead of taking a pill, though, I squatted and stopped my ordinary thoughts to concentrate my attention on the pulses along the meridians of the Diamond Being. I rode the pulses up and then brought them down the scale. In addition, I placed both elbows against wood beams and let the pulses reverberate from shoulders to elbows to fingers. I discovered that when I held my breath a few seconds after my inhale, I could set up a metronome of pulses. If you know when, you know how: exactly how is a matter of individual experimenting, since each person's channels develop a little differently. In truth, diagrams of the channels are approximations meant to guide the intuition. Although these channels have no physical equivalents in the nervous system, they exist nonetheless; the ancients, unhampered by scientific facts, discovered the "subtle body" and tried to understand it. I could use my arm for shooting again whenever I followed this procedure. If I picked up the bow and tried to shoot right away, though, the arm hurt.

The oddest reality I've been forced to consider since the healing of my arm is not that I was able to shoot my bow after this Seiki-Jyutsu, or pulse "healing" work, but that the best doctoring is not about health, it's about the transition from the rational to the spiritual attitude toward treatment. With the spiritual attitude, the patient becomes a partici-pant in the healing process, responsible for improvement. The healer shows the patient the way, pulse by pulse. I don't believe in magic, and yet I wouldn't trust my life to any system of treatment that didn't acknowledge the life force.

1 7

A SUNRISE
CONCLUSION

Certain beliefs about the power of the Diamond Being are clearer in sacred moments or on sacred occasions. Such beliefs are appropriately private, yet they draw us to public festivals. One frosty October morning, I was awakened at 5:30, and Larry, one of the other students, made sure I didn't fall back asleep. We were to attend the sunrise ceremony at the old pueblo on San Geronimos' Day.

Parking and walking areas for tourists are strictly regulated around this, the oldest continuously inhabited community on the mainland. Piñon fires scented the festival grounds, where food and craft merchants had set up booths. Most tourists wore ski clothing, but occasionally I'd see them in traditional Indian getup or western wear. The Native Americans milling around wore jeans and plaid wool jackets, while those on the ceremonial running track wore only loin cloths and sneakers. Most of the runners were older men with large bellies, flaccid arms, and broad chests. There were more teenage boys running than middle-age adults. We walked about, for although the sun was up, it hadn't appeared over the breastlike peaks of Creation Mountain.

Larry and I were drinking coffee when the master and

the tall, wily old American monk arrived. We heard drums and chanting as the races were to begin. The runners should have been shivering and freezing, but they weren't. I didn't have to ask the master what it was that kept them warm; their posture was evidence enough.

A Western nutritionist might look at the old men's bodies and lament their lack of exercise and proper diet. Cultural blindness is akin to ignorance. The fact is that these ceremonial racers showed, to the informed eye, mastery of many of the same disciplines as my Japanese teacher. The lessons had been passed down for almost as long at the pueblo as in the temples of Kyoto.

I knew the kind of strength in those bellies and arms, aware of it now as clearly as I'd overlooked it ten years before. Then, I wouldn't even have speculated on the similarities between Native American running, the Eastern stillness in motion, and the art of shooting arrows from horses. Now I was finding parallels in my own tradition. At my cabin I had a book on the medieval kabbalist Abraham Abulafia, by Moshe Idel of the Hebrew University in Jerusalem. Abulafia's four main principles were much like the ones I had spent weeks learning: (1) breathe in a fixed rhythm, (2) balance your head on your spine, (3) focus on the human internal structure, (4) make a spiritual sound while exhaling.

Listening to the drums and singing at the sunrise ceremony, I couldn't help but think of the similarities among the chants of all tribes. The drums fed the spirit and urged the breath and posture to fill the wells of ki. With this power the runners sped along the track lined with spectators, oblivious to the cold and to the crowd. In a few minutes they were out of our sight. We wandered about, and the air was sanctified with tradition where I stopped to admire a recently carved Indian bow of osage orange wood. The bow was thick and resilient—a short twenty-two-inch arrow would have deadly power when shot with this much spring.

Indian bows were made to be carried in a quiver draped over the shoulder. Asians had to keep their longer bows in saddle sheaths to accommodate the length and curves. The Native American shot his short bow by placing his left hand over the arrow and pulling back under it with the right. When I handled the bow at the display booth I could tell why. The tension caused by the sinew backing was stored more in the handle than in the limbs. The left hand would aim, quickly following the eye movements, and the right hand would snap the string back. Coordination was more important than muscles, since the bow was meant to be shot quickly. A quick pull meant that balance on the horse was not jeopardized. And since Native Americans originally rode without saddles and stirrups, balance was critical. This short bow, I figured, would be ideal for riding down animals or enemies at breakneck speed.

Watching the contemporary warriors circle back through the cold motivated my desire to try the Native American bow and arrow on horseback. Here, running had been turned into a spiritual pursuit of power. I could feel the form it took in their bodies. Even more so, I could sense the presence in mind that commanded their movements, even to the point of intuiting the way this presence would handle the short bow on a swiftly moving horse.

As the price of the bow at the booth was over $400, and

the seller warned me that osage wood bows might crack, I decided to stay with my modern bow even if it was eight inches too long.

The ceremonial arena filled as the sun rose, illuminating the thirty-foot greased poles that awaited the climbing antics of the Native clowns. The clowns were painted with black-and-white stripes and wore corn stalks in their hair. A brisk business was being done at the booths in the crafts area during the lull in activities. At one booth I discovered an unusual silver chain made by a Zuni grandfather. I had with me a Tibetan medallion of a dragon designed in the form of a figure eight. The dragon symbol represented the animistic demons that underlie Tibetan Buddhism. I'd worn the dragon on a short leather tie, and when I hung it from the longer chain that let it reach my heart, I received a ki jolt quite unexpectedly. The monk who had introduced me to the Zuni man suggested that the piece was a talisman, pointing out that the ruby eyes and turquoise mouth were powerful gems. I had a different view of his insight. Both the figure eight and the diamond form describe the positions of the wells of ki. This was especially evident in the medallion, with the dragon's mouth sitting where the tanden would be. In kabbalistic tradition a similar diagram calls the ten points sapphires. This diamond-shaped diagram, known as the Tree of Life, represents the shape of the internal being. I believe that any concentration on this shape can generate the ki, given the right circumstances.

This ceremony certainly aroused the presence in mind that made people more aware of hidden dimensions of life. It was a serious day of communion at a very serious place. We shared respect for the true target, that mysterious self attuned to the old, transcultural teachings. My father would not have understood them, but I have a suspicion that his father would have. For a person's presence in mind remains the crucial missing part of our contemporary life. We must learn to walk with it all over again.

The master explained that a walker in the Sea of Origin is the traveler in history who, although he can't see into the remote past, knows that it provides him with both the flow and the pattern of this moment. Origin is present if the Sea becomes the screen on which his actions take place. As the screen provides perspective, what isn't graceful or in harmony with the Sea disturbs and confounds us.

So, it's the 1990's and I am upon a horse shooting arrows using styles from both sides of the world. I can shoot at a faster speed using the Native American style, more accurately with the Mongolian, and at greater distance using the Japanese. I, myself, am the son of East European Jews who hadn't used bows and arrows since biblical days. I remained intrigued by a resemblance between the Zuni grandfather and the Japanese Zen master. This sunrise, they, the runners, I, and many others, had come together for a ceremony celebrating the Sea of Origin that seemed so omnipresent when I was riding against the backdrop of Creation Mountain.

The experience I needed to duplicate the ceremonial runners' intensity was right here in an open field. Out of curiosity, I tried the Native style of bow shooting. I quickly discovered that this kind of archery required more strength in the left forearm than I could muster more than a few times. Becoming accurate required a completely different push-pull and pointing method than I'd learned: a difference in technique, yet one still had to be attuned to an arc to feel the trajectory for the arrow. The arc needed was more like that of throwing a horseshoe at a peg. With this arc the arrow drops much more rapidly, an advantage for hunting. One other advantage is that the arrow can be shot along a wider horizontal sweep, or even back over the shoulder. I could get a shot off even if the horse slanted against the line of the target because of my ability to pivot a short bow.

I moved closer and closer to the target, confirming my suspicion that the archer's range is limited when using the eye-over-the-left-hand style. The reason is that the right hand doesn't draw back a long arrow along an arc. It's the difference between a rifle and a pistol, the long arrow acting like the rifle's barrel. I found that using the Native American style forced me to track the target ahead of me, looking outward rather than inward to the form. Despite this variation, something remained the same in the three styles I knew. The constant was—despite the horse's motion—to trust in the something above and beyond the ordinary, make-certain self. It was necessary to understand that the ceremony of this other self, our Diamond Being, existed in every culture. I was discovering a faith in the harmony between the deep self and the world's flux.

For further reading. . .

ZEN AND THE PSYCHOLOGY OF TRANSFORMATION

The Supreme Doctrine

by Hubert Benoit; Introduction by Aldous Huxley
ISBN 0-89281-272-9 • $12.95 paperback

While Western psychology tends to focus on problems rather than possibilities, Zen seeks to activate true human potential. This classic work advocates an integration of Western psychological thought and the wisdom of Zen.

"...the ancient Zen masters would have given Benoit their imprimatur. He has understood their secret and made it his own. He invites us most searchingly to do the same."
London Times

TAO AND T'AI CHI KUNG

by Robert Sohn
ISBN 0-89281-217-6 • $12.95 illustrated paperback

It is the unification of spiritual principles, emotion, and intellect in conjunction with movement that constitutes Taoist Yoga, or T'ai Chi Kung. This book is the first to discuss the deeper secrets of energy development, including the concept of rooting one's body in the earth's energy and connecting of this energy to specific acupuncture points.

THE MEDITATOR'S GUIDEBOOK

Pathways to Greater Awareness and Creativity

by Lucy Oliver
ISBN 0-89281-360-1 • $7.95 paperback

A teacher of meditation explains the basic process of meditation, describing its benefits and pitfalls, and shows how patient observation, concentration, and volition can bring calmness, power, and insight to the practitioner.

YOGA: MASTERING THE SECRETS OF MATTER AND THE UNIVERSE

by Alain Daniélou
ISBN 0-89281-301-6 • $10.95 paperback

A fully authentic account, based entirely on original Sanskrit sources, of the methods of Yoga in its different forms, including techniques of the more challenging "left-hand" paths. Of special interest is the author's insight into the unique requirements and capacities of today's aspirant and the specific practices appropriate to Western students.

"...the foremost living interpreter of Hinduism...his books are remarkable for their clarity and scholarship."
Interview Magazine

THE DIVINE LIBRARY

A Comprehensive Reference Guide to the Sacred Texts and Spiritual Literature of the World

by Erich Keller
ISBN 0-89281-351-2 • $12.95 paperback

As a guidebook to the diverse streams of spiritual wisdom, this directory to the primary religious literature of past and present cultures defines more than 120 entries, with bibliographic references to available editions, translations, and commentaries.

THE BUDDHIST HANDBOOK

A Complete Guide to Buddhist Schools, Teaching, Practice, and History

by John Snelling
ISBN 0-89281-319-9 • $14.95 paperback

This is the first book to provide an overview of Buddhism worldwide—the different schools, concepts, interpretations, teachers, and organizations, from its early history, meditation practices, and festivals through the Westward migration of Buddhist thought. It also includes a Who's Who of Buddhism from a modern Western perspective.

CRYSTAL AND DRAGON

The Cosmic Dance of Symmetry and Chaos in Nature, Art, and Consciousness

by David Wade
ISBN 0-89281-404-7 • $14.95 illustrated paperback

Exploring the interplay of form and energy, David Wade takes us on a journey through the world views of successive ages— from Plato's conception of the ideal form and the ancient Taoist philosophy of change to the modern scientific view of structure embodied in the laws of physics—showing how prevailing perceptions about the nature of the universe are reflected in the art of their times.

PSYCHONAVIGATION

Techniques for Travel Beyond Time

by John Perkins
ISBN 0-89281-300-8 • $10.95 paperback

For centuries, visions and dream wanderings have been used by people in cultures around the world to tap into sources of inner guidance and bring them a greater understanding of themselves, their creative force, and their environment. In *Psychonavigation*, John Perkins brings you step-by-step techniques to attract this inner guidance for help in making decisions and developing creative solutions to challenges in every area of life.

THE BLACK BELT MANAGER

Martial Arts Strategies for Power, Creativity, and Control

by Robert Pater
ISBN 0-89281-295-8 • $10.95 paperback

A consultant to Fortune 500 companies, Robert Pater applies the strategies of some of the most sophisticated martial arts to the challenges of corporate management. He shows how martial arts principles can help you influence others by controlling yourself; sustain inner calmness under attack; harness commitment to a mission, and translate minimum effort into maximum gains.

"...packed with ideas for improving control over one's energy. Swimming against the current just doesn't work. It is much more effective to channel energy and alter the course of events as they unfold. Pater's techniques work."
John Chapman, General Manager, General Electric Co.

CENTERING

A Guide to Inner Growth

by Sanders Laurie and Melvin Tucker
ISBN 0-89281-050-5 • $7.95 paperback

Offering a unique system of meditation techniques for those who want more out of life, *Centering* helps you increase personal learning power and healing energy, discover new talents within yourself, and ultimately learn how to live at ease in a stressful world.

WAYS TO BETTER BREATHING

by Carola Speads
ISBN 0-89281-397-0 • $9.95 illustrated paperback

The author, who studied and taught for many years with the pioneering movement teacher Elsa Gindler, shows how the quality of breathing determines the quality of life. Whether you use breath consciously—as in teaching, the performing arts, heavy labor—or would simply like to learn basic techniques to alleviate the pressures of stressful living, her program of gentle breathing exercises will bring more vitality and fulfillment into your life.

CREATIVE VISUALIZATION

by Ronald Shone
ISBN 0-89281-214-1 • $9.95 paperback

It is widely recognized that people can create transformations in their lives by generating powerful imagery. This book explores the practical application of visualization techniques in business, sports, and personal development, showing you how to use creative visualization to realize life goals.

To order directly from the publisher, send a check or money order for the total amount, payable to Inner Traditions, plus $2.50 shipping and handling for the first book and $1.00 for each additional book to:

Inner Traditions, P.O. Box 388, Rochester, VT 05767

Be sure to request a free catalog.